Second Chances

Receiving the Gift of Life

By

Jeffrey R. Lueders

Jim,
Thanks for your support of organ and tissue donation. Enjoy the book. May God Bless.
Jeff Lueders

RAGGED EDGE PRESS
SHIPPENSBURG, PENNSYLVANIA

Excerpt from "The Final Act," on page 67, used with permission from the *Cincinnati Enquirer*, John Johnston.

Sheree Starr, mother of my organ donor, Brandon Burress, gave approval for information and copies of Brandon's medical chart and other records, which I received from the University Hospital in Cincinnati, to be used in this book.

Portions of an article, written by Dr. David J. Stevens, were printed with permission in chapter 4, pages 31–32. The article were taken from *Decision* magazine, October 1996; © 1996 Billy Graham Evangelistic Association.

This Ragged Edge Press publication
was printed by
Beidel Printing House, Inc.
63 West Burd Street
Shippensburg, PA 17257-0152 USA

In respect for the scholarship contained herein, the acid-free paper used in this book meets the guidelines for permanence and durability of the Committee on Production Guidelines for Book Longevity of the Council on Library Resources.

For a complete list of available publications
please write
Ragged Edge Press
Division of White Mane Publishing Company, Inc.
P.O. Box 152
Shippensburg, PA 17257-0152 USA

Library of Congress Cataloging-in-Publication Data

Lueders, Jeffrey R., 1955-
Second chances : receiving the gift of life / by Jeffrey R. Lueders.
p. cm.
Includes index.
ISBN 1-57249-219-8 (alk. paper)
1. Lueders, Jeffrey R., 1955- 2. Organ donors--United States--Biography. 3. Donation of organs, tissues, etc.--Case studies. 4. Heart--Transplantation--Patients--Biography. I. Title.

RD129.5 .L84 2000
362.1'783'0922--dc21
[B]

00-062684

PRINTED IN THE UNITED STATES OF AMERICA

This book is dedicated to my wife, Debbie, whose love and faith are a constant inspiration, and to Brandon Burress, whose 15-year-old life was cut short on June 26, 1989, a hot and muggy summer day.

All my life's a circle
Sunrise and sundown
The moon rose through the nighttime
Till the daybreak came around

All my life's a circle
But I can't tell you why
The seasons spinning 'round again
The years keep rollin' by.

–"Circle," the late Harry Chapin

Contents

Illustrations

Introduction

Getting a second chance wasn't easy

For most people, turning 40 is a milestone, complete with a birthday celebration. That birthday came for me on January 21, 1995. For me, it was a birthday I never thought I'd celebrate. In 1989, two Cincinnati cardiologists and a cardiac transplant surgeon gave me six months to live. My life seemed devastated. I had idiopathic congestive cardiomyopathy. The prognosis was bleak. It was late 1984 and early 1985. In short, the doctors said my heart muscle was damaged beyond repair and was functioning at less than 10 percent. A heart transplant was the only treatment that could save my life. That would come June 27, 1989. For four long years before the transplant I barely clung to life.

I continued to work as a public relations account executive for one of Cincinnati's largest advertising agencies and do some freelance work. Tired, weak and short of breath, I found it hard to climb even the smallest set of stairs or walk from room to room at home and at the office, and I had always used the stairs at the office.

Before my illness, my life was active: work, basketball two nights a week at Gamble-Nippert YMCA, and racquetball once a week. I dated but still lived at home with my mom. The meals were great and the laundry was cheap. My time was occupied with the yard work, taking Mom to the store and helping out around the house. We got along well. I loved her and she loved me.

Dying had never crossed my mind before the diagnosis. Dying was for grandparents who had lived long and fruitful lives, whose time on this earth was gone. My father had died on April 15, 1977, when I was only 22, also from heart disease. He had two severe heart attacks and died at 54. After being sent to the Indiana University Medical Center early in 1985 for evaluation, I remember praying one night to him that these "were the best of times, these were the worst of times." (Charles Dickens' *A Tale of Two Cities*, Greenwich House, 1982, p. 35; first edition published in 1859.)

I can only imagine how people with terminal illnesses like cancer or AIDS view life and death. Days become moments and each moment is precious, for life itself is precious. It is something to hang on to until the very end. Dying had crossed my mind but it wasn't time yet. I had prepared for it, though. My friend, Mark Minges, a funeral director from the west side of Cincinnati where I live, and I discussed pre-need funeral arrangements but that was all, even though my grandfather, years before, had purchased a six-grave plot at Spring Grove Cemetery. I was determined to live. On days in which some of her energy was sapped, Mom used to say how nice it must be for the people who are in Spring Grove Cemetery. "Their cares and worries are over."

Several years ago, Bill Wallace, one of my liver transplant friends who lives on the west side, said in an interview with the media that "most people will never understand what it means to face death and then have a second chance." Those of us who have had second chances know exactly what he is talking about.

I developed a bad case of bronchitis shortly after Thanksgiving Day in 1984. Two weeks of antibiotics did little to help. It was a cold, gray Saturday, December 10, 1984, when our family physician, Dr. William Heil, saw me for the second time. I was sweating profusely. The temperature outside hovered in the 20s. It was almost winter. He sent me to the emergency room at Good Samaritan Hospital in Cincinnati. From there I went to the cardiac step-down unit at the hospital. My two cardiologists, Dr. David Tondow and Dr. Brian Skale, told me I had idiopathic congestive cardiomyopathy. It was Christmas time in 1984 and I knew I was very sick. From Good Samaritan Hospital I was sent to Indiana University Medical Center in Indianapolis. Dr. James Hager confirmed the diagnosis but no mention was made of a heart transplant. The heart transplant program in Cincinnati didn't begin until late 1985. I was so sick in Indianapolis for the month I was there, including Christmas and New Year's that my diet consisted of jello, cottage cheese, and soft drinks. I went from 197 pounds to 159 pounds in three weeks. That was when I began to blame God.

From my point of view, God could have prevented the whole thing from happening. I found it very hard to go to church. My faith wavered. Blaming God just seemed like the natural thing to do. Then the realization came to me that these things are allowed to happen. I guess I'll never know why. But I couldn't help questioning God and the more I sought an answer, the more I discovered there was no concrete answer. I'd look around at my neighbors and friends and see their lives going smoothly. No problems. No sickness. No worries. I became cynical and skeptical of everything that went on around me. It's very easy to have a lot of faith in God and your church when everything is going well. But I was turning away from God and my church just when I needed them most. Eventually, my faith was restored and I returned to church. Still, three years after I was diagnosed, I had to fight with Social Security for disability insurance. It was a long road to regaining my health and my faith. (See chapter 4)

My deterioration was quick; sometimes I wished for death, even though earlier I had cherished life. Living was not worth the agony. I'd get up at 7 A.M. and arrive at work by 8 A.M. By 5 P.M. I dragged myself home on the bus, ate supper, read the paper, and went to bed. I could no longer play basketball on Friday nights and Saturday afternoons. Racquetball, too, was impossible. I went to California for three weeks in the fall of 1987. The change of climate did me good but my heart was still failing. I tried desperately to play basketball. But five minutes or less was all I could tolerate. For all intents and purposes, my life as I had known it was gone. I hated the world, God, and what my illness was doing to my mom. She did not know what to do. I worked until late 1987 when I went on disability and Medicare.

Mothers have a way of making you believe in yourself with strong beliefs and undying faith. Mom, and my grandmother, until two years before her death in 1990, were both steadfast in their belief that something good would come of this. I, of course, was doubtful. But I guess deep down inside of me I must have believed it and began to realize that maybe they were right. In spite of my doubts – in God and my cardiologists – I became more positive and reached out to Mom and Grandma like never before in the past. I was not the strong one and I needed their help and guidance. I reached out to them and they were always there, always faithful. One of Don McLean's early songs is called "And I Love You So." One of the lines goes something like this: "The book of life is brief. And once a page is read. All but love is dead. That is my belief." I had their love and their faith.

From 1985–1988, I became depressed. I wanted to cry but I did not. The tears would not come. I had trouble sleeping. Walking up a few stairs tired me. So did walking. The energy was just not there. I knew I was going to die. It was just a matter of time.

Having heard and read a lot about heart transplants, my new cardiologist, Dr. Walter H. Herzog, helped me hold on with several medications. My own heart was diseased and worn out. I sought a third opinion from another cardiologist, Dr. Robert Toltzis of University Hospital in Cincinnati. University is one of two heart transplant centers in Cincinnati, the other being Children's Hospital Medical Center. This was in September 1988. The same day of my visit with Dr. Toltzis, I received a call from Julie Collins, the clinical transplant coordinator with the cardiac transplant program at University Hospital. The process of being listed had begun. Even though I held Medicare and a health insurance supplemental policy from Blue Cross and Blue Shield, the cardiac transplant program was not Medicare certified. I had to "spend down" my assets and go on Medicaid to get the heart transplant.

In September 1988, I met the cardiothoracic surgeon who began the heart transplant program at University Hospital in 1985. His name was Dr. David Melvin. Dr. Melvin had an easygoing disposition and a Tennessean drawl that made me take a liking to him immediately. He drove a Jeep Cherokee, I think. His salary would have permitted an expensive luxury or sports car. But he was unlike any physician I've ever met.

He now works in research with mechanical heart assist devices at the University of Cincinnati Medical Center and occasionally recovers hearts for LifeCenter, the local organ recovery agency. He returned to school at Ohio State University to study mechanical/biomedical engineering. He is currently working on his doctoral thesis. I still see him in the hospital and Medical Sciences Building occasionally and at our support group's annual picnic and Christmas party. He readily admits he took a 90 percent pay cut to continue in research. But he is happy and relaxed and loves his new work. He once told a *Cincinnati Post* reporter, in the days when he was transplanting hearts that "I went from being a very young 43 to a very old 47." The pressure to run the cardiac transplant clinic, evaluate potential recipients, recover hearts, and do 85 percent of the transplants for five years was enough to make a young man old. For relaxation of both mind and body Dr. Melvin, with the help of his sons, put in a new driveway at his Hyde Park home, brick by brick (he now lives in Loveland, Ohio, just outside Cincinnati). (See chapter 4) He occasionally recovers hearts for LifeCenter, the local organ recovery agency in Greater Cincinnati. To put it simply, I love the guy. He and the transplant team saved my life and gave me a second chance. You don't forget individuals like that.

After about a month of tests and being cleared by a social worker and the financial counselor, my case went to the Transplant Selection Committee. If approved, the Ohio Solid Organ Transplant Consortium also had to give its blessing. By February 1989, I was officially on the list, happy but anxious. Six months to a year was the approximate time I was told I would probably have to wait. Just holding on long enough until a heart became available was my goal. I was given a pager and sent home. I returned monthly for blood work and evaluation. The people at the cardiac transplant clinic were great: Julie Collins, the clinical coordinator, Jarlath Black, the clinic nurse, and Kathy Gosney, the social worker. They were like family to me. And so were the recipients I met who had already been transplanted. They gave me the courage, determination, and fortitude to go on.

I visited Charlie Ashcraft at his home in Cold Spring, Kentucky. He was the first to have a heart transplant at University Hospital on December 17, 1985. He had worked at the General Motors assembly plant in Norwood prior to his transplant. I was number 73. When I asked Charlie what to expect, he simply unbuttoned his shirt and showed me the scars. "All in all it's not so bad," he said. The foot-long zipper scar, the two small incisions where the chest tubes were inserted, and the barely visible scars from the wires placed inside to be used, if necessary, for defibrillation to restore normal rhythm, made me a little apprehensive but that was all. Unfortunately, Charlie died in 1990. I gave a short eulogy at his funeral.

As it is with all organ transplant candidates, the wait for my heart was unbearable. It was very stressful. Every time the telephone rang or my pager went off, I thought a heart was available. But the minutes turned into hours, the hours into days. I tried to live as best I could with renewed faith. My faith did return and I thank God it did. For without a lot of family, friends, colleagues, and fellow parishioners praying for me, I know I would not have made it. The great thing about God is that you may give up on him but he never gives up on you. God was going to be there for me and I'm glad I finally accepted his help.

Sometimes I'd lie awake at night and listen to my weak heart barely beating and think that soon somebody else's heart would be beating inside me. I was amazed and a little scared and sad, for I knew only somebody's death could save my life.

A year and a half after the transplant I began working in public relations for LifeCenter. I am the public affairs manager. To see firsthand how organs are recovered in the operating room and know how organ allocation works was a career change I am very proud I made.

Tom Tressler, former director of organ procurement at LifeCenter, left the organization early in 1996 after 11 years. It was time to move on. He now works as regional director of the Make A Wish Foundation in Greater Cincinnati. But to have seen him make half a dozen telephone calls to see if we were going to accept an organ from another center, watching the adrenaline flow, and the expression on his face when he knew a life was going to be saved, never lost its appeal. Now, to see senior transplant coordinator Wendy Valerius get the initial call from a hospital with a potential donor, and then see her leave for the hospital as fast as she can, is a never-ending drama that may have a happy ending or may result in no donor at all. To see Katie Evers, manager of clinical services, smiling from ear to ear when she gets word that the heart she brought in from Dayton, Ohio, several days ago is functioning superbly in a 35-year-old father of three, makes the job seem worthwhile. Mark Sommerville, assistant director and media spokesman, is out there every day educating the media, the public and professional community of physicians, nurses and clergy so that they can do their job better in the request process. David D. Lewis, our executive director, who oversees the administration and day-to-day operation of LifeCenter, leads us.

There is sorrow too. It is frustrating and sad when transplant coordinators Missy Holliday or Ruth Ann Hanto or Teri Mestrich or Wendy remove a name from the local waiting list because that person has died. They never get used to it. The rewards are when they meet the recipients leading fairly normal lives. They can see in their faces the gratitude and thanks that make the job invaluable.

And I hope in some small way, that the tasks I tackle make a difference. It's been more than 12 years since the transplant. I didn't think that love would ever come my way. The subtle discrimination by employers that I experienced when trying to return to work was evident in dating too. "You really need a heart transplant?" "You had a transplant? You look so good." Common comments I got used to hearing. I had pretty much resigned myself to being a bachelor for life when I began dating a lovely lady I had known for about two years. After a month, the magic seemed to be there. I gave her a cassette recorded by the late Jim Croce to play one Friday night. I had it set on "I'll Have to Say I Love You in a Song." I was never much for showing emotion. But I knew I loved her and she loved me. Her name is Debbie. She was a medical secretary to two transplant surgeons at University Hospital. And now works for one of the associate deans of the University of Cincinnati College of Medicine, Dr. Robert Highsmith. We were married May 20, 1995.

Marriage does not scare me in the least. What does worry me, though, is not knowing how long I'm going to live. A few heart transplant recipients in the United States have lived more than 15 years. One, Tony Huesman, an acquaintance, was transplanted at Stanford University Medical Center in 1978. He lives in Dayton, Ohio. Another, one of Dr. Christian Barnard's early patients in South Africa, recently died after having his heart for 23 years. What is Debbie going to do when I die? I guess that's where God takes over. Rather than worrying about when I'm going to die, I think I'll just live for the moment. I don't discuss it with her because it just upsets her.

For now, I am happy. I still play basketball one night a week at the YMCA. I also walk and work out on the exercise equipment at the Y. I make the most of each and every day. I try to live each day as if it were my last. And I often tell high school students when I lecture, that even if I were to die tomorrow, I've still had more than 12 years that without a heart transplant I would not have had. I have participated in the U.S. Transplant Games (an Olympics every two years for organ recipients) in Indianapolis in 1990; Atlanta in 1994; Salt Lake City in 1996; and Ohio State University in Columbus, Ohio, in 1998.

Life is something that should never be taken for granted. Coming close to death was something I was neither afraid of nor worried about. Maybe that's only partially true. I was prepared for it. Without a heart transplant I would have died. I was ready. God was not ready for me. In Richard Bach's *Illusions, The Adventures of a Reluctant Messiah,* he writes through one of the characters, "Here is a test to find whether your mission on earth is finished: If you're alive, it isn't." My life is complete and I'm happier than I've ever been.

This book pays tribute to the love and generosity of donor families. Without them, there would be no second chances for those of us who suffer

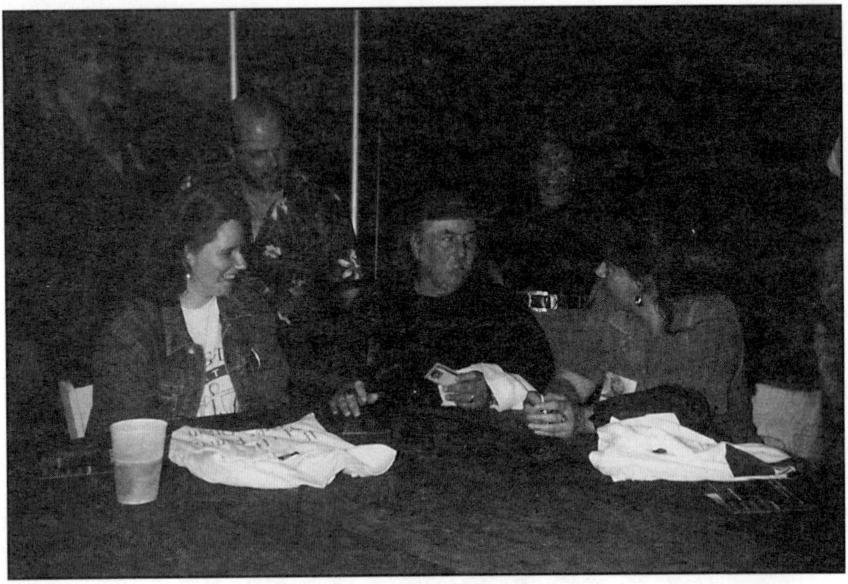

Backstage with David Crosby

After a Crosby, Stills and Nash concert on June 5, 1996, at Cincinnati's Riverbend Music Center, the Coalition on Donation (the national group promoting organ and tissue donation) members and volunteers met with David Crosby, a liver recipient. *Left to right:* Elizabeth Flynn, community affairs and public relations director of the Regional Organ Procurement Agency of Southern California (ROPA); Theresa Eisenberg, former education coordinator of the Cincinnati Eye Bank; Howard Nathan, coalition president and executive director of the Gift of Life Donor Program; David Crosby; Laura Monken, former administrative assistant for LifeCenter; and Edie Sorvino, former executive director of the coalition.

Photograph © by Mark Sommerville

end-stage organ failure. They and many, many other donor families make a decision that saves and enhances the lives of as many as 50 individuals. Their decision to donate organs and tissues comes at a time when they suffer their greatest personal loss. But through the tragic death of their loved one they know that their loved one lives on in others. Through this, they find peace and solace. Saying "thank you" to these families seems so inadequate. But we do so each day we are alive. By the grace of God and through their generosity and caring, we endure with our second chance.

This book also pays tribute to transplant recipients and their families, showing the courage, determination, and fortitude we have in staying alive long enough to receive our "gift of life" and in the care of this "gift" as we lead normal, healthy, productive lives.

Our families, donor families, friends, transplant friends, and the healthcare professionals who continue to care for us form a special bond. We are an extended family.

On June 5, 1996, I met David Crosby of Crosby, Stills and Nash at a concert at Riverbend Music Center in Cincinnati. They performed with Chicago. Some colleagues and I from LifeCenter and the Cincinnati Eye Bank went backstage to meet Crosby who had a liver transplant on November 20, 1994. Crosby has volunteered his time and energy to help promote organ and tissue donation. We were all handing out brochures promoting organ and tissue donation at each gate that night for the concert. In fact, the band's 47-city tour that year promoted organ and tissue donation through the national efforts of the Coalition on Donation. Crosby is a great spokesman. Sitting across from him, we were talking about organ transplants, immunosuppressive medications and donation. His wife, Jan, found out I had had a heart transplant and asked me to go backstage. I met Crosby and his young son who was born after Crosby's liver transplant. Referring to our medication and follow-up care, he said to me, "You know what I'm talking about." I will never forget those words. I had a bond with David Crosby because I had a heart transplant and he'd had a liver transplant.

Section I

My Story

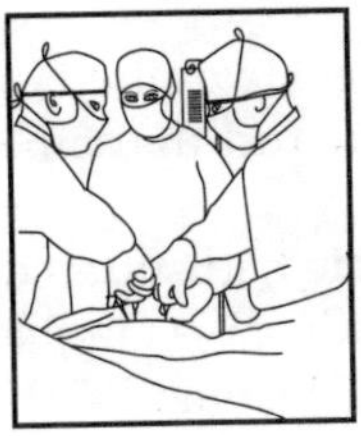

1

This one's for you, Dad!

Though my dad, Robert Lueders, died at the relatively young age of 54, I learned a lot from him. He taught me to switch hit and shoot baskets when I was three or four. I played Knothole baseball for eight or 10 years. I was never a standout player. I was only an average player. But that was OK with dad. For several years he was my coach. I attended my first Cincinnati Reds game at Crosley Field in 1961. The Reds played the Philadelphia Phillies.

Aside from sports, Dad took me to Indian Guides at the YMCA. I have belonged to the Gamble-Nippert YMCA for more than 35 years thanks to dad, for he insisted I learn about mind, body, and spirit (John 17:21). Dad served a number of years on the Y's Committee of Management.

As I grew up, I played basketball in grade school, junior high, and high school. As in baseball, I was not a standout. I was pretty good, though. Dad's one lesson in life: It isn't whether you win or lose, but how you play the game. Unfortunately, to this day, I find it a difficult lesson to follow. I still play basketball one night a week and still have that same competitive edge I had growing up. Maybe I expected more of myself than dad did. He played baseball at Western Hills High School in Cincinnati from 1936–40. He was an average player, too.

In the 1930s and '40s, Dad ushered at Crosley Field. He saw the Reds lose the '39 World Series to the Yankees in four games. But he also saw them beat the Detroit Tigers in a thrilling seven-game series in 1940. I remember Dad telling me about pitcher Johnny Vander Meer, the only major league pitcher to throw two consecutive no-hitters (June 11 and June 15, 1938 at Crosley Field and Ebbets Field in Brooklyn), perhaps the greatest sporting feat of the 20th century. He also spoke of other great players he saw play: right fielder Ival Goodman, pitchers Bucky Walters and Paul Derringer, first baseman Frank McCormick, catcher Ernie Lombardi, and manager Bill McKechnie. We enjoyed the Reds' back-to-back World Series Championships in 1975 against Boston and 1976 against the Yankees.

Dad had a good sales job and even worked as an accountant for one of Cincinnati's largest advertising agencies. He needed just a few credits to graduate from the University of Cincinnati in business administration. I think my grandparents and my mom were disappointed he never finished college. It didn't bother me at all.

Dad was a loving man. He cared about Mom and me. He exalted in our triumphs and helped us through our failures. And we did the same with him.

He died of a massive heart attack on April 15, 1977. He had suffered his first heart attack in May 1976. The last time I saw him alive was in the cardiac intensive care unit at what is now Mercy Franciscan Hospital-Western Hills in Cincinnati. We talked about the Reds' loss the night before. Jack Billingham had pitched. That was our good-bye. I cried when he died the next day. Not very long. It was one of the few times I cried in my adult life. I was 22. I was sad. Mom grieved. But you pick up the pieces and go on with life.

Some of my happiest memories of Mom, Dad, and me were a September 1975 vacation to Colonial Williamsburg in Virginia. It was a short week, but I still remember the mountain air and view in West Virginia. I remember leaving one of our suitcases in the parking lot at the Patrick Henry Inn in Williamsburg. We discovered it was missing somewhere in the mountains near Charleston, West Virginia. Dad stopped at a pay telephone, called the hotel and a week later the suitcase arrived at our house in Cincinnati with everything in it. Someone had kindly turned it in to the front desk.

I remember the first theatre production I attended. Dad and I went to Cincinnati's Playhouse in the Park and saw Jason Miller's Pulitzer Prize-winning play, *That Championship Season*, about the reunion of a high school basketball team who had won the state championship 25 years earlier. The performance got me hooked on theatre. I have since written three one-act plays.

Dad seemed to me to be carefree and happy, with a constant smile on his face. He was optimistic about the future, saying it would take care of itself. There is seldom a day that goes by when I do not think about him. I know he's looking down on me from heaven. Even though he wasn't alive to see me receive a heart transplant and a second chance at life, I know he was there in spirit. He attended church frequently and reminded both mom and me to keep the faith. Shortly before he died, he told my grandmother that he thought living to 54 was all right. I think he knew he was going to die or he wouldn't have said that. My one regret is not telling him I loved him more than I did.

The lessons I learned from dad are still important to me. I remember him for the way he lived his life. I am a better man because of him. And though he is dead, I know he is always with me in spirit. I know we will meet in heaven. Thanks for everything, Dad! I love you.

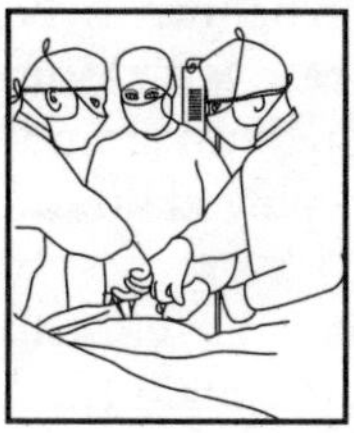

2

Family and heart transplant

An organ transplant is very difficult for the recipient. And as long as you remain on a waiting list you are always referred to as a potential recipient. Every 16 minutes a new name is added to the national waiting list, which grows by about one thousand names each month in the United States. More than 72,000 people are on the national waiting list. On average, 13 people—men, women, and children—die each day in the United States because an organ is not available. More than 270 people are waiting for organs in Greater Cincinnati where I live. But I am one of the lucky ones. For more than 12 years I have lived with the heart of a young man who was 15 when he died. Words can hardly express my gratitude to this young man and his family. So I try to live each day as if it were my last. There simply is not enough time in each day to do everything I want. There are not enough hours in the day to do everything I'd like to do.

Sometimes, in the back of mind, I have this notion that it will not be so bad dying young, not living to become a senior citizen and maybe a burden on my family. I never think about dying. Only about living. I received my master's degree in English on June 12, 1998. I started my studies when I was very near death and completed it after my heart transplant. I began this book in April 1995 and finished it in April 1998. As I look out my office window each day, I marvel at the surroundings. The birds and trees and sky and clouds and sunshine and rain. Life. They all symbolize life and remind me about all the brave recipients who came before me, paving the way, and those who came after me. Some are still living. Some have died. We are all like one extended family, with the same motivations and the same zest for life. We are miracles of modern medicine. Each night I say a silent prayer for all the organ and tissue recipients in the world. We are unique. Each of us received a precious gift.

Before I became a modern miracle, though, I was on the waiting list. Each of the 61 organ procurement organizations (OPOs) in the country maintains a local waiting list. Your medical condition, geographic location, and length of stay on the waiting list are determining factors in receiving an organ. This wait is equally difficult for your family—in my case, my mom, Adele, and my grandmother, Mildred M. Motsch.

From 1985 to 1989 I was not even on a transplant waiting list. By the time I was on the list, my grandmother had fallen and broken her hip. Even though she was in her late 80s, she made a rapid and heroic recovery. Mom and Grandma possessed a deep faith. It never wavered. Though my grandmother died in 1990, eight months after my transplant, she played an important role in my recovery, as did my mom.

Mom was born in 1921 on McMakin Avenue in Winton Place, close to Spring Grove Cemetery in Cincinnati. She was nicknamed Mitzie (pronounced Mitezie) because she was so small. My grandparents, her mom and dad, were born and raised in Winton Place. The family moved to Westwood on Cincinnati's west side in 1922. In the early 1940s they moved to a rural home in Bridgetown on Werk Road with two and a half acres. One summer during World War II, almost every Sunday when Mom would sun herself in the backyard, a young Air Force pilot in a P-15, or something similar, would fly over her house and tip his red cap to her. She would wave back. Several Sundays he flew very low and between the houses. "Neighbors wondered who that 'reckless' kid was," says Mom. "That day he flew so low, my father suggested I better stop sunning myself." Mom recalls that later though, Grandpa would just come in and get me if I wasn't outside for the pilot on Sundays, saying something like, "Mitzie, your pilot friend is out there again."

In the early 1960s, Grandma and Grandpa retired to a smaller home in Cheviot. In 1977, they came to live with Mom and me. My dad, Robert, had died of a massive heart attack on April 15, 1977. My grandfather was in the lumber business, supplying the lumber for large construction projects like Shillito's (now Lazarus). So mom basically grew up on the west side of Cincinnati. She graduated from Western Hills High School in 1939. That same year, she began her studies at the University of Cincinnati (UC). She remembers the tuition in those days was about $1,500 for four years. She graduated in 1943 and for the next 15 years was director of several day care centers in Cincinnati. She had a blind date with Ed Jucker, who was also a UC student and went on to become head coach of the Bearcats basketball team, leading them to two straight national championships in 1961 and 1962. She remembers being in a coffee shop on the campus of Miami University in Oxford when the Japanese bombed Pearl Harbor. "It was so quiet in there," she recalls, "you could hear a pin drop."

She enjoyed travel very much. For six straight years she and a high school and college friend traveled by train to New York City. "To wake up in a Pullman car and see the sun coming up over the Hudson River was so beautiful," she says, remembering those days as if they were last week. They walked through Harlem.

Other travels took her to Hawaii, Mexico, the Virgin Islands, Puerto Rico, Haiti, the Caribbean, and the Bahamas. She never got to go to Europe and still longs to travel there. She met a man in Hawaii who asked her to stay and teach school. In the Virgin Islands, she was also asked to stay and teach school. Mom was very attractive in those days. She still is. Her first true love, Charlie Givens, graduated in her class from Western Hills High School and went to UC as well. He enlisted in the navy in World War II; he was killed at Guadalcanal in the South Pacific.

Grandma was born in Winton Place as well in 1899. Her father came from Germany and immigrated through Ellis Island. Grandma had seven brothers and sisters, though the two youngest, Tillie and Frieda, died when they were infants. Her maiden name was Goosmann. Her father, Richard, was a baker and owned several St. Louis flat buildings and bungalows in Winton Place. My great-grandmother, Josephine, lived off this income until she died at the age of 95.

Three of Grandma's brothers were quite successful and wealthy. Her youngest brother, Richard, who was to go into the bakery business with his father, died of typhoid fever when he was in his early 20s. He is buried at Spring Grove Cemetery. Charles, her oldest brother, was one of Cincinnati's first radiologists and he also taught at the University of Cincinnati College of Medicine. Mom always spoke of their mansion in Wyoming and the servants they had. Dr. Goosmann probably was exposed to huge amounts of radiation and that is probably what killed him. Grandma finished the 11th grade at Hughes High School. Both she and her younger sister did not finish school because the teachers made them very nervous. Grandma learned English grammar, punctuation, history, math, chemistry, and physical science from Charles. Mom says she never made a grammatical error in her life. I never heard her make one grammatical mistake. She worked as a secretary for Charles at his office but had to quit. One day, she told a potential patient on the telephone that Dr. Goosmann had office hours by appointments only. Charles overheard this exchange and corrected her, saying it "was by appointment only." That night at home she told her mother Charles made her too nervous. The next day she promptly told him "Momma says I don't have to work for you because you make me too nervous." Charles shrugged his shoulders and said if that was the way she felt, she could quit. He was just doing it for her own good. He probably missed her efficiency around the office after she left. I was born at Deaconess Hospital where Dr. Goosmann was on staff. One of the nurses who took care of my mom after I was born said that all the nurses were scared to death of him. Charles and his wife, Iva, died in the 1960s and are buried at Spring Grove Cemetery.

Her next oldest brother, Fred, had a very successful machine tool business in Harlington, Texas. He did quite well before, during, and after the war, adapting new products to meet a changing America. His son-in-law,

Spencer Booze, took over the business when he retired. He died in the 1960s and is buried in Spring Grove Cemetery, not far from where he grew up.

The brother that Grandma was closest to was Herb. Herb was a star athlete at Woodward High School and went on to play football, basketball, and run track for the University of Cincinnati between 1910 and 1914. The UC backfield and one lineman in those early years were known as the Goose, the Fish (after a guy named Fishbach, the quarterback), and the Bear. Bear was Teddy Baehr, an offensive lineman who got his picture taken once in front of a Stutz Bearcat, and is possibly where the school's nickname was derived. Well, that's one of three stories of how they became the Bearcats. Herb was the fullback/halfback. Anyway, Herb missed very few homecomings in UC's history until he was in his early 90s. The drive from Florida home became impossible and he didn't like to fly. He always came to Grandma's for a meal when he was in town. Grandma used to carry the basketball on the streetcar for him when he played in high school and college. She was always real proud of that. Herb graduated from UC in 1916 with a degree in civil engineering. He became assistant to the president of the Singer Sewing Machine Company in New Jersey. He and his wife, Ann, and their daughter, Joanne, lived in Elizabethtown, New Jersey. Herb actually designed and patented the first portable Singer sewing machine. Mom used to have one of the original models until about 1995.

Grandma loved baseball and was a Reds' fan early on, listening to the games on radio and later watching them on TV. She knew a lot about baseball, from the game itself to the players. She once tried to explain the hit and run to Mom after they saw it on TV.

Grandma was closest to her youngest sister, Marjorie Gronauer. She was only a few years younger. They had a small farm in Bridgetown, raising a few animals, including horses, and crops. Her husband, Clifford, worked in a factory all his life. Her two children, Cliff and Ginny, grew up with my mom. Mom is very close to Ginny. They are like sisters.

Grandpa died of a stroke in July 1984. Grandma died in the winter of 1990. Both of them are buried at Spring Grove Cemetery.

In a 1991 book, *Organ and Tissue Transplantation: Nursing Care From Procurement Through Rehabilitation* by M. K. Gaedeke Norris, former education director at LifeCenter, and Mary Anne House, both authors stressed the necessity for family support and cooperation. In order to achieve this cooperation and continued support, the transplant process must be understood. For that reason, my mom was included in the educational process, including the sharing (with me) of a three-ring binder called *Living With Heart Transplantation,* produced by Sandoz, a subsidiary of Novartis Pharmaceuticals. She was part of most of the pre- and post-transplant question-and-answer sessions.

Patient and family education during the evaluation, say the authors, is to inform your family of the transplant process, its risks and benefits. In that way, lines of communication are open throughout the entire process. "In addition," say the authors, "a precedent for patient and family involvement is established that prepares them for the transition to post-transplant teaching."

I was lucky to have both written and individualized personal contact with Dr. Melvin and Julie Collins, the clinical transplant coordinator at University Hospital, regarding test results, procedures, and checkups. Meetings with the social worker, Kathy Gosney, and Lynne Powell, the financial counselor, were also very helpful.

Before I went on the waiting list for a heart at University Hospital, I was very depressed and very, very sick. There was no chance I would get better. My options were death or a heart transplant. Death did not seem like an option at the time. I initiated a second and third opinion about my cardiomyopathy. The heart transplant program at University Hospital was only a little over three years old when I was listed. I liked the surgeon, Dr. Melvin, who ran the program. I found his Tennessean drawl relaxing. I felt very comfortable with him, before, during, and after the surgery. I liked Julie Collins, Dr. Melvin's nurse, Jarlath Black, Kathy Gosney and Lynne Powell. I felt comfortable with them. Perhaps my second chance was going to come after all. There remained, though, much uncertainty and stress. I didn't realize how competitive it was to get an organ transplant.

The competition for improving my health with a new heart really started five long years prior to my being listed. Sometimes I felt so bad that I wished I would die. A dark, haunting depression came over me. As I watched the joy and happiness in the faces of other people, like my friends, fellow workers, and the people in my neighborhood, I retreated into my own little world, blaming God for my illness. I stayed away from church. Mom went and prayed for me. I lay in bed on Sunday mornings, often too tired to get up, but also so angry at God for allowing this to happen. I wondered how people with terminal illness faced the pain and suffering day in and day out. Mom kept the faith. Grandmother kept the faith. I did not. Friends at church kept the faith and prayed for me, as did friends and neighbors. The depression came and went. I wrote three short one-act plays, submitting them to contests and readings.

Being an avid basketball and racquetball player, I found myself always on the sideline, always a spectator, not even able to take a walk most days. Exercise of any kind made me tired and weak. I felt helpless and alone. I was not. Mom and Grandmother were always there. Still, I couldn't sleep. It was like a nightmare that would never end.

"It was disturbing news," mom says, of my diagnosis of cardiomyopathy in late 1984 and early 1985. "It was upsetting and it was worrisome.

I thought you were going to die. I was just beside myself. At that time, there was no mention of a heart transplant."

Barely a month after my diagnosis, Mom felt a lump in her left breast when she took a shower. The day she went to the doctor and had the tests, Grandma and I prayed all day. The surgeon, an old high school and college friend of Mom's who had lived across the street from her on Werk Road, asked her permission to remove the entire breast if the lump was cancerous. Mom agreed. The day of the surgery Grandma and I just prayed that it would only be a lump removed. It was the whole breast.

"I was very upset with the initial news," says Mom. "My grandmother (paternal) had died of breast cancer. And of course, I was afraid I was going to die." But through it all, her faith in God was steadfast. "Through your sickness and my breast cancer, I kept the faith and knew that the Lord would take care of us. Your grandma kept the faith and prayed every single day for both of us." Today, Mom is 79. She looks 10 years younger. Many people think she is much younger.

In 1985, Grandma fell in our living room and broke her hip. After her surgery and recuperation, she had to move to an assisted care nursing home called Riverview. It is one of the United Church of Christ's homes. She was rehabilitated and began walking about six months after her fall. Three years later she had a debilitating stroke that left her bedridden and unable to speak very much. "I explained to her about your heart transplant," recalls Mom. "I'm not sure she comprehended everything I told her but I think she knew you were doing fine. In her heart, she knew. She's watching over you today."

"But from 1985 until she died in 1990, I never knew from day to day how Grandma was going to be." Mom visited her at least twice a week and talked to her every day until the stroke. I always visited her on Sunday with Mom. "Grandma had serious heart problems too, going into cardiac arrest on several occasions. It was uppermost in my mind that something was going to happen to her too." Mom's worries seemed endless.

When I finally had to relinquish my job in 1987, with a large Cincinnati advertising agency, I felt sure the end was near. But in September 1988, my reprieve came when I sought a second opinion. After a few tests and telephone calls, it seemed I would be evaluated for a heart transplant. Dr. Robert Toltzis (mentioned in the introduction) was the cardiologist's name. I remember very well his attractive nurse who administered several of the tests. She even told me about a very beautiful young patient with long, dark hair who had graduated from Purdue. She also had cardiomyopathy.

It was at this point I believed the medical system would come through for me. I had finally found my miracle. Then the question of who would pay for the transplant had to be addressed. Even with Social Security Disability and Medicare, I had to go on Medicaid because the cardiac transplant program at University Hospital was not Medicare-certified for heart transplants. It became Medicare-certified for heart transplants a year later in 1990. Medicare wouldn't pay for the transplant in 1989. I learned later about the Ohio Solid Organ Transplant Consortium. Nobody in Ohio can be turned down for an organ transplant because they cannot pay. Renal transplants and dialysis have been covered under Medicare since 1972.

Officially, I went on the cardiac transplant waiting list at University Hospital on February 10, 1989, at 1:49 P.M. The cardiac transplant program at University Hospital had to approve me as well as the Ohio Solid Organ Transplant Consortium in Columbus, Ohio. This happened between October 10, 1988, and February 10, 1989. To be put on the waiting list for an organ transplant with the United Network for Organ Sharing (UNOS), tests and evaluations have to be done by the transplant program before approval is given.

Being on the cardiac transplant waiting list for five months and then the transplant itself were traumatic. "It was stressful for everyone, but especially you," says Mom. When I ask her if she thought I'd get better, she replies, "I constantly prayed for that. I knew with a heart transplant you'd be able to lead a normal life again.

"Your cardiologists from 1984–1988 did not seem interested in exploring the option of a heart transplant for you. I thought when you sought a second opinion about your cardiomyopathy it was the best thing you could have done. And it was. Nobody else seemed to be interested in getting you on the transplant list. I admire you for taking it upon yourself to explore this option."

The second week of June in 1989 I received an afternoon call about 2:30 P.M. from Julie Collins saying not to eat or drink anything. "We may have a heart for you," she said. I didn't know if it was a local donor or if the organ would be flown or driven to Cincinnati from another city. Julie had trouble reaching me because I did not have my pager on. I was scolded in fact. About an hour later Julie called back to say the family did not want to donate their loved one's organs, including the heart. I understood. I was disappointed and sad. I thought that might have been my only chance. The hard truth was that someone had to die so that I could live. But I did become tethered to the pager from that day on.

Both Mom and I still remember vividly the 3 A.M. telephone call from Dr. Melvin on June 27, 1989. It was hot and muggy when we left the house about 3:45 or 4 A.M. Mary Ellen Betz, my second cousin and a nurse (actually she's a registered nurse and also holds bachelor's and master's degrees as well as a doctorate in nursing, and teaches nursing at the College of Mount Saint Joseph in Cincinnati), picked us up. Dr. Melvin wanted me at the hospital by 4:30 A.M. I was sitting on the couch in our TV room in my boxer shorts and a T-shirt when I took the call.

"I was a nervous wreck," recalls Mom about that morning. "I had to take an Ativan I was so nervous. And I'm sure you were very nervous." Actually, I was very surprised at myself because I was not nervous but extremely calm. Maybe I was just in my own little world, just concentrating on what was in store for me during the next 12 hours or so. I remember driving to the hospital with Mom sitting in the back seat. At that hour of the morning there was little traffic. We arrived at the hospital fast. As we drove, Mary Ellen was talking about taking her nieces and nephews, two boys and two girls, to Paramount Kings Island the day before. I just kept thinking to myself that she was talking about having fun the previous day at Kings Island, an amusement park, and I was going to get a new heart. I'm afraid I didn't share her laughter and enthusiasm.

"The whole ordeal was mind boggling," says Mom. "It was hard for me to understand and hard to realize this was happening to us. My question to God, of course, was 'Why is this happening to you?' I should not have been questioning God. You are not to question the Lord. He knows what he is doing."

Dr. Melvin had told me to check in at the emergency room of University Hospital. When we arrived, at about 4:25 A.M., I told the nurse at the admissions desk in emergency that I was there for a heart transplant. She immediately called upstairs to let Dr. Melvin know I had arrived. Then I was taken to x-ray by a nice, jovial, middle-aged man who was either the technician or an orderly. My next destination was to a room on the cardiac intensive care unit (CICU) where I put on a hospital gown. I remember the anesthesiologist and several other doctors began to hook me up to more tubes and wires than I'd ever seen before. Blood was drawn. A myriad of tests were run and I really did not have much time to think about the whole ordeal because it all happened so fast. I later found out there was a delay in the recovery of the organs from the donor. The operating room was ready at 11:30 A.M. on June 27. I remember being wheeled down to the operating room (OR) on a gurney and telling the anesthesiologist I wasn't very sleepy. That was the last thing I remember until I woke up approximately 12 hours later in the CICU. I actually arrived in the OR at 12:30 P.M. and the procedure began at 1 P.M.

That was the last thing I remember until waking up with a respirator irritating my throat. It was removed about 24 hours later. The sternum saw had made a 13-inch incision in my chest. The chest retractor spread my rib cage wide open so the surgeons could remove my diseased heart and sew in the new one. Chest tubes and wires were placed inside my chest cavity as well, the wires to be used if defibrillation was needed to restore normal rhythm. It was not needed. The metal sutures and my breastbone were wired back together. My chest felt a little uncomfortable. But two weeks later I walked out of the hospital and began taking walks at home. In several weeks I was shooting baskets at the YMCA. In two months I was back doing freelance writing and working out on the exercise equipment at the YMCA. Cardiac rehabilitation followed as well. Participating in sports was fun again. I was no longer just a spectator. Life was fun again.

Following are the recollections of Mary Ellen Betz regarding the 13-and-a-half hour ordeal of my heart transplant. Mary Ellen reflected upon her pieces of memory surrounding my surgery.

I came to get you about 3:45 A.M. and we dropped you off at the ER entrance. Your mother and I parked the car in the garage and came in. They took you to "wherever" to prep you and we went up an elevator to a waiting room where they had told us to go. As I recall, the donor family was already there – but we had no idea who they were; they were just "other people" in the waiting room and their anxiety was evident – tearfulness and pacing. We were sitting in an arrangement of chairs separate from them.

We were in the waiting room a while before the relationship between the donor family and us became apparent, and I recall that they initiated the questioning to us. At some point in time, I think after they had left, your mom and I were approached by the clinical transplant coordinator from the transplant team who indicated how highly unusual it was for the two families to be in the same waiting room. I don't remember what prompted her (Julie Collins) to approach us, but perhaps it was comments to her by the donor family. I do remember my telling her that it had been uncomfortable at times on both sides.

To back up a bit – before the donor family left – I know there was some exchange of information. They asked your mom for your name and address and she gave it to them with some hesitation. It was a very awkward point as I recall. I know we expressed condolence and appreciation to them and they expressed hope to us for your surgery being successful.

Your mother and I were then called in to see you and we went in for maybe 15 minutes. The donor family was asked to leave with the understanding you were going to the OR. We had breakfast in the hospital cafeteria and your mom took her medicines. Then we returned to the same waiting room. We were told there was "a delay" and you had not gone to the OR yet and we went back to sit with you.

You were in the cubicle directly across from the area you were in postoperatively. I would estimate we sat with you for one to two hours. There were nursing and medical personnel in and out of the room the entire time. You were awake and talked with us during this time. When they finally came to take you to the OR, we left and went to a room with two beds they had assigned to us. It was close to the waiting area and we sort of drifted between that room and the waiting room. We were kept well informed of the progress of the surgical procedure and your status throughout. At some point, we went to the cafeteria for lunch, and then back to the waiting area. Once the surgery was completed, I left your mother there and went home to your house to let the dog out, then to my place to check on my company and my parents who had come to Cincinnati to have dinner with Jean (Mary Ellen's sister-in-law) and the kids (her nieces and nephews). Wayne, my husband, took them all out and I returned to the hospital to see you.

I remember the number of IV (intravenous) solutions and tubes and the nonstop care the nurses gave you. Your mother and I were both in reverse isolation gear and you were awake but lethargic. I think I visited you twice while you were in the hospital. After we visited that first evening, I took your mother home.

Mom says Mary Ellen explained the transplant procedure to her in terms that were easily understood. "I didn't know how to react to his (the donor's) family, and I guess they didn't know how to react to me," recalls Mom. "I knew who they were. We were the only ones in the surgical waiting room. They came up to me and asked if I was your mother. They assumed who we were, that we were there for your transplant. We stood talking and it was a very sad situation. All of us were crying. Since I was upset, it did not register with me at first who they were. I know Brandon's grandparents were there. Everything turned out for the best. Dr. Melvin said you came through the surgery fine."

That afternoon, when I came out of the recovery room, Rev. Glen Halbe, associate minister at our church, Pilgrim United Church of Christ, came to the hospital. "He came back the same evening because we were still there," recalls Mom. "It was a nerve-wracking experience to say the least. I would never like to go through anything like that again."

Rev. Cal Klumb, our senior minister, also visited me often. I received so many cards and well wishes from friends and my church family that I hardly had enough space for them in my room.

The type of heart transplant I received was orthotopic, meaning basically that my anterior atria and ventricles were completely replaced. The posterior atrial walls of my donor's heart were connected through surgery, to the remnant cuffs of my atria, and the aorta and pulmonary artery connected end-to-end. The blood is slowly warmed through the cardiopulmonary bypass circuit. As the heart is gradually allowed to fill and stretch, a spontaneous rhythm often begins. I am not sure if low-voltage defibrillation was used to initiate a regular beat.

I was on the operating table and monitoring was established via a central venous line and an arterial line. My chest area was prepared with iodine solution and draped with sterile towels and sheets. According to the operative note by Dr. Melvin, when they opened my chest at 1:20 P.M. with a standard median sternotomy, my heart was greatly enlarged, much like a football minus the tips on each end. It was also sluggishly contractile, meaning it was hardly contracting at all. I was placed on cardiopulmonary bypass (with two venous cannulas posteriorly in the right atrium extending into each vena cava and arterial line high in the ascending aorta) after establishment of full heparinization, timed so as to have me stable on bypass at the expected arrival time in the OR of the donor heart. I went on bypass at 1:49 P.M.

The donor heart arrived in the OR and my body temperature had cooled appropriately. The ascending aorta was then clamped just below the arterial line after tightening venal caval tapes and allowing the heart to empty as much as it would. My heart was excised, dividing the aorta and the pulmonary artery just above their valves and both atria just posterior to the tricuspid and mitral valve. Both the atria and both great vessels were trimmed so as to present a smooth circular or elliptical surface for suturing. This involved resection of the major portion of both atrial appendages.

The donor heart was removed from its cold container. Its temperature was 4°C. The left atrium was prepared by joining the four pulmonary veins and resecting redundant irregular corners. The right atrium was prepared by extending the inferior vena caval orifice superiorly parallel to the atria septum for about 2 cm and then directing toward the right atrial appendage obliquely until a sewing margin approximately equal to that of my right atrium had been achieved. A 3-0 polypropylene suture was then started at my left superior pulmonary vein and Brandon's left atrial appendage, and continued circumferentially until the left atrium had been connected.

Starting in the mid-septum, the right atrium was similarly connected. The tip of the left atrial appendage was amputated and the left atrium was cannulated with a large bore cannula for infusion of cold saline. Cold saline infusion was begun at 200 ccs per minute. My body temperature was beginning to rise. A 3-0 polypropylene suture was started at the left extremity of my donor's heart across the posterior wall to the right side. The other end of the suture was continued across the anterior wall, using suction to aspirate the egressing cold saline from the aorta for visibility, but allowing the aorta to remain full for expulsion of air. When the connection was completed, the suture was tied as I was placed in the Trendelenburg position, head down on a table inclined at about 45 degrees from the floor with my knees uppermost and legs hanging over the end of the operating table. With an aspirating #20 needle just through the suture into the aorta and the blood pressure lowered by reduction of the pump flow, the aortic clamp was slowly released as blood was aspirated. The pump flow was gradually increased and the heart observed for fibrillation. Cold saline infusion was stopped at the completion of the aortic connection, after aorta unclamping and the cold line removed with ligation of remaining atrial appendage using 0 silk. Using a similar technique, the pulmonary artery was connected with 3-0 polypropylene.

My warming was completed. The connection was checked for leaks, the heart was filled, and the connection was checked again for leaks. Cardiopulmonary bypass was successfully terminated at 3:30 P.M. Protamine sulfate and methylprednisolone were administered. Cannulas were removed; two large chest tubes, two atrial and three ventricular pacing wires were placed in my abdomen, along with any needed permanent epicardial pacing wires. The wound was closed using interrupted 0 silk for pericardium, interrupted #6 wire for sternum, continuous 0 Vicryl for presternal fascia and the linea alba, continuous 2-0 Vicryl for subcutaneous tissue, and skin staples for the skin.

:ocedure ended at 4:30 P.M. and I was out of the OR by 4:45 P.M. irst to the post-anesthesia care unit (PACU), then to the cardiac :are unit (CICU) in stable condition. I had tolerated the procedure weı..

I was extubated a day later and put on cyclosporine, prednisone and azathioprine postoperatively to prevent rejection. On July 3 I had the first of many, many endomyocardial biopsies and I was then transferred to the cardiac stepdown unit. There I received rabbit anti-thymocyte serum (RATS), a rejection serum that made me extremely sick and gave me severe headaches for three days. It was used postoperatively to delay the onset of rejection and is used in conjunction with other immunosuppressive medications. The remainder of my hospitalization, until release on July 10, was uneventful, according to my discharge summary. But to me, the transplant was anything but uneventful. The only pain I had after the surgery was where my sternum had been cut. The incision measured 13 inches long. I entered the hospital 14 days earlier, very near death. I was about to leave, a new man, strengthened by the gift of someone I did not know. The experience was traumatic.

A week after the transplant, my mom brought a newspaper clipping to me in the hospital. Organ and tissue donors always remain anonymous, but my donor family stayed in the surgical waiting area of the hospital when I received my new heart. As mentioned earlier, they introduced themselves to my mom and Mary Ellen. Julie Collins did not want both families to meet. The clip was the death notice of my donor. Today, it is framed and hangs along with photos of my donor in our bedroom. His name was Brandon Burress. He was 15 when he was hit by a car on his bicycle and killed riding home from summer football practice at Blanchester High School. The young man who hit him was a former student and football player at Blanchester who was going to Miami (Ohio) University in the fall.

Three of Brandon's goals prior to his death were to get good grades, play varsity football, and learn how to drive when he turned 16 in March 1990.

I called his grandparents on Thanksgiving Day 1989. I thought the call would be hard. It wasn't. They were glad I called. We have met, we occasionally talk on the telephone, and we exchange Christmas cards. Brandon's mother, Sheree Starr, sent me a photo of him when he was 14. Kneeling in his football uniform with his hand on his helmet, I often wonder where he'd be today if he had lived. The family has also sent me three other pictures of Brandon: when he was five, eight, and 15. One of the last photos of Brandon is taken of him at 15 in his football uniform. The pictures are a constant reminder of just how blessed I am. Not a day goes by when I don't thank God, Brandon, and the entire transplant team for giving me a second chance. Brandon is buried in Graceland Memorial Gardens, a Milford, Ohio, cemetery. I visited his grave for the first time on April 23, 1995.

A transplant recipient has five major hurdles to overcome before, during, and after the transplant. First, you have to be evaluated and listed at a transplant center, in my case, at University Hospital's cardiac transplant program. Second, a donor must become available. Third, you must survive the transplant itself. Fourth and fifth, you must fight to prevent rejection and infection for the rest of your life. A simple case of the flu or a cold that goes untreated could pose a serious health risk and even death if it develops into pneumonia or other complications. You have to be careful of any kind of cut or scrape.

Immunosuppressive drugs combat rejection for as long as you have your transplant. These drugs are chemical agents that cause the human organism not to produce antibodies that normally fight off foreign material in the body. The production of these antibodies needs to be thwarted or suppressed in order to permit the acceptance of the donor heart.

The immune system, according to the manual mentioned earlier, *Living With Heart Transplantation*, is made up mostly of white blood cells known as lymphocytes. To better understand how the system functions, this is what happens when a virus invades our body. Outside the human body, a virus is little more than a bundle of genetic information. Once it enters the body, it multiplies and takes on a life of its own. The macrophage, a cell that circulates in your body and helps fight off foreign invaders, acts somewhat like a foot soldier and is the first line of defense. It surrounds the foreign matter, like a new organ, and tries to digest it. When it is unable to suppress most of the invaders by itself, the macrophage sends out an "SOS" to the next line of defense.

Helper T cells answer this call. After identifying the invader, the helper T cell travels to the spleen and lymph nodes where it gives the command for other types of white blood cells in your body to be produced and recruited. The killer T cell, a very important foot soldier, is a type of white blood cell that responds to the command of the helper T cell by killing off the virus. Killer T cells also destroy cells in the body that have become cancerous.

The B cell, another important component of the immune system, is found primarily in the spleen and lymph nodes where it does its part in fighting the battle against the virus by following the command of the helper T cells and producing an army of antibodies. The antibody is a powerful chemical weapon. When a virus or other infectious agent invades the body, the antibody rushes to the source of the infection and renders it harmless.

When a new heart is transplanted, the antibody views it as foreign matter or an invader and can cause your body to reject it. That is why the body must be suppressed with immunosuppressive drugs.

When the virus has been halted successfully, the suppressor T cell commands the immune system to call off the attack so there are fewer killer T cells available to destroy body cells and less B cells to produce antibodies against the invader.

The memory cell is a specialized cell that helps your body "remember" how the invasion was stopped, so that it can respond to future attacks on your immune system in the future by the same or similar enemies. The memory cell is produced during the initial stages of attack.

My medication list today includes cyclosporine, azathioprine and prednisone, three immunosuppressive medications. Cyclosporine is an oil-based medicine that prevents rejection by decreasing specific cells that recognize the newly transplanted heart. Azathioprine prevents rejection by decreasing the number of white blood cells in the body. Prednisone is a steroid hormone that prevents rejection by decreasing the inflammatory response of the body.

While cyclosporine, azathioprine, and prednisone work to inhibit the action of helper T cells and other cells which cause adverse reactions, such as infections, they do have some very serious side effects. Cyclosporine does not depress the function of the bone marrow, the place where many cells are produced. However, as it suppresses the immune system, you become more susceptible to colds, the flu, and other harmful viruses. It can also cause kidney dysfunction, hand tremors, body hair growth, high blood pressure, swollen or bleeding gums, and headaches.

The side effects of azathioprine include an increased risk of infection, nausea and vomiting, mild hair loss, decreased white blood cell count, as well as other blood abnormalities.

Prednisone may cause swelling of the face, hands or ankles; stomach irritation that could lead to bleeding ulcers; weight gain due to an increase in appetite or fluid retention; heightened risk of infection due to the suppression of the immune system; "steroid-induced" diabetes; skin changes including slower healing of bruises, more delicate skin, rash or acne on the face, chest and back; increased hair growth; muscle weakness; osteoporosis; fluid imbalance; mood swings; and cataracts.

Additionally, after the transplant, I was on verapamil, dipyridamole, potassium chloride, antibiotic, nystatin, antacids, and a stool softener. Verapamil, a calcium channel blocker, works to affect the movement of calcium into the cells of the heart and blood vessels, relaxing the vessels and increasing the supply of blood and oxygen to the heart while reducing its workload. Dipyridamole and Ascriptin® prevented the platelets from clumping together and sticking to artery walls, narrowing the artery and reducing the flow of oxygen. I only took dipyridamole for about three years because it gave me terrible headaches. Potassium chloride was a potassium supplement. I no longer take this medication. Antibiotics are used to treat infections. It was used as a preventative medication for the first several years. I no longer take this medication. Nystatin was an antifungal medication used to treat fungus infections in the mouth. This I no longer use either. I also take an antihypertensive.

On July 10, 1989, 14 days after my heart transplant, I left University Hospital. I started walking a mile or two a day, both outdoors and at the mall. I felt like a new person. The first place I stopped on the way home was Skyline to get a 3-way chili. A year and a half later I began a job in public relations at LifeCenter. Today, (as mentioned earlier in the introduction), I am public affairs manager. I have a lot to be thankful for.

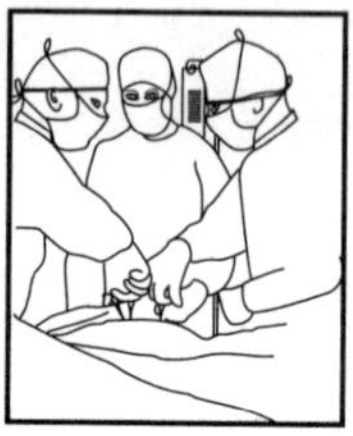

3

King of hearts

I first met Dr. David Melvin in September 1988, when I was being evaluated for a heart transplant at University Hospital in Cincinnati. I was impressed not only with his abilities in dealing with patients like me facing end-stage organ failure, but in his kind, compassionate manner. I knew right away that I trusted him to do my heart transplant. His manner was casual—from the way he talked to the way he dressed to the way he always made me feel at ease. But I knew hidden under this demeanor was a perfectionist and a surgeon who was somewhat hyperactive, all for the good of his patients. He was intense and thorough. He did everything at full-speed. He was brutally honest with me. I remember him telling me, in his Tennessee drawl, shortly before I went on the cardiac transplant waiting list at University Hospital on February 10, 1989, "Jeff, you have a 50/50 chance of making it through 1989 without a heart transplant. Those aren't very good odds." I didn't need to be talked into having a heart transplant. It was the only thing that would save my life.

And so began my odyssey. The doctor/patient relationship has become a genuine friendship. It is going strong today. My wife, Debbie, and I are very close friends with Dr. Melvin. He and his wife attended our wedding in 1995.

Dr. Melvin grew up in Bradford, Tennessee. "We called it a town," recalls Dr. Melvin. "It was not really a city. Here in Cincinnati it would be a village or a crossroads."

Dr. Melvin was born in 1942, the son of high school teachers. He has a brother, Billy C., who is 17 years older. His father, William Clifton (W.C.), taught agriculture, machine shop, economics, and political science. His mother, a substitute teacher, taught art. She was also a gifted painter herself. Dr. Melvin's brother, Billy, left for World War II when Dr. Melvin was barely three months old. "He's more like an uncle than a brother," says Dr. Melvin affectionately. Billy lives in Missouri with his wife. He has two sons and a couple of grandchildren. Dr. Melvin's father died at age 90 and his mother in her early 80s. "My parents were in their 40s when I was born," says Dr. Melvin. "But my dad kept teaching school, mostly at Bradford High School where my brother and I went, until he was almost 80. He persuaded a series of school boards that he was still up to teaching."

So what got Dr. Melvin interested in medicine?

"That's a hard question to answer. I started out liking math and physics. I was ending my junior year of college at Union University in Jackson, Tennessee, and I had a girlfriend who had been injured in an automobile accident. I was hanging around the hospital, as she was getting better. And I just kind of said to myself, 'I wonder if I could do this?' I opened the college bulletin to see if it was too late to get all the prerequisites for medical school. In a lot of ways, I guess it was a whim. I think it was a correct one. But just kind of a 'why not?'"

And so Dr. Melvin began medical school at the University of Tennessee. He liked it very much. He finished second in his class of about 80, graduating in 1967.

He met his wife, Sue, on a blind date when he was in medical school. She was a nursing student. Sue worked at the University of Tennessee Hospital and also at Duke University in the intensive care nursery.

The Melvins have four sons: Mark, 32; Alan, 29; John, 23; and Peter, 20. Mark is a computer consultant in New York City for Lotus Notes. He lives in New Jersey. Alan is a civil engineer and works with his father at CardioEnergetics, a biomedical research firm he (Dr. Melvin) founded in the late 90s. Alan has become a mechanical and biomedical engineer. John graduated in 1998 from Emory University and attends law school at the University of Cincinnati. Peter is a junior at Emory University, majoring in math and physics. He may go to medical school.

Dr. Melvin says he chose surgery because he was interested in mechanical devices and engineering applications to medicine. "I thought I would be a lot closer to implementing these applications in surgery than I would be anywhere else in medicine," he says. "The conception of treating the physiologic problems of patients sometimes involved mechanics and the use of engineering-type devices. That made sense to me."

Dr. Melvin began his general surgery residency training at Duke University in Durham, North Carolina, in 1968 and spent two years there. He was very interested in cardiac surgery. From 1970–1972 he was a clinical associate at the National Heart and Lung Institute. He then completed his general surgery residency at Cornell-New York Hospital in New York in 1975. Dr. Melvin says the general surgery program at Cornell was great experience. "In general surgery you see a wide variety of things," he recalls vividly. "But also being in the middle of New York City gave the experience even more diversity in a lot of different ways."

At the University of Michigan in Ann Arbor, Dr. Melvin completed a fellowship in thoracic surgery in 1977.

After the fellowship at the University of Michigan, he wanted to go into an academic program to teach and also to operate. "At that point," says Dr. Melvin, "if you're a surgeon and you don't operate a good deal in your first few years, you don't develop the skills. It is probably not as important to keep it going at a hard pace but you really have to—at least I did and I think most surgeons do today. I found a place, the Wichita branch of the University of Kansas. It was a combination of a private practice and academics. They let me do some teaching and some research and I had a very busy clinical practice. It turned out to be some of both worlds but probably not the best of either world. But I learned a lot and worked with good people."

At about this time, Dr. George Callard, whom Dr. Melvin knew at the National Heart and Lung Institute called him to see if he'd be interested in joining Cardiovascular and Thoracic Surgeons Inc. in Cincinnati. Dr. John Flege had begun this practice after his residency when he returned to Cincinnati in 1969 to become chief of cardiac surgery at The Christ Hospital. He had graduated from the University of Cincinnati College of Medicine in 1954. Dr. Flege completed his surgical residency at UC in 1963. He did his fellowship in cardiothoracic surgery in London, England, at Hammersmith Hospital from 1963–65. Dr. Callard had joined him from the University of Virginia in 1971. Dr. Edward Dunne of Vanderbilt joined in 1980. Dr. Creighton Wright, Dr. Jim Wilson, and Dr. Donald Mitts also joined Dr. Flege.

"I met with the group," recalls Dr. Melvin, "and after about a year John called me up and asked, 'Are you really happy out there on the Plains?' I decided I would come to Cincinnati and take another look at their program. I decided that as much as I liked the academics, research, and teaching that I really liked operating more and this was an environment in a very, very good group. I joined the group purely in private practice in 1979 without much hope of working in the academics. But as things worked out in the three years after I joined, we were over at University Hospital organizing the cardiac surgery program and we became academicians."

Dr. Flege organized the cardiothoracic surgery department at University Hospital with him being professor and chairman of the division. Dr. Melvin and the rest of Dr. Flege's group came along. "After about two-and-a-half or three years the group decided we needed a heart transplant program," says Dr. Melvin. "I certainly wanted to be part of it," recalls Dr. Melvin, "partly because of my interest in mechanical heart assist devices and a heart transplant program offered the opportunity to apply these devices. It was fascinating. I went to the University of Pittsburgh and spent time at Stanford, two of the country's largest heart transplant programs. I did experimental transplants in the laboratory. Then I became the heart transplant surgeon at University Hospital. My partners assisted but I wound up doing most of the heart transplants. In the beginning, for the first few transplants, I would call up one of my partners and say, 'Could you open for me while I go get the heart and help me sew it in?' or 'Would you like to do it and I'll help you sew it in?'"

Dr. Melvin, Dr. Dunne, Dr. Flege, Dr. Callard, and Dr. Mitts were part of the team of cardiac surgeons that performed the first heart transplants at University Hospital on Charles Ashcraft (December 17, 1985) and Bill White (January 1, 1986).

But Dr. Flege and the rest of his group returned to private practice after the first two heart transplants at University Hospital. Dr. Melvin remained and ran the cardiac transplant program as program and surgical director until 1990.

"My understanding of why John (Flege) left the heart transplant program at University Hospital is that once the cardiac surgery program in general was started, of which transplant was a part, the medical school asked John to stay, saying they needed him full-time. He basically said no, that's not the agreement I started under and if I'm going to be full-time anywhere it's going to be at Christ and Jewish Hospital. So he bowed out. I am still good friends with John and all my former partners. At that point, heart transplant was staying here and I really had an interest in teaching. Sooner or later I knew I was going to end up principally doing research and University Hospital and the Medical Center is the place to do that. And Dr. Tom Ivey came to head cardiothoracic surgery."

From 1985 to 1990, Dr. Melvin toiled many, many long hours to make the cardiac transplant program the success it is today. As of September 2000, more than 295 heart transplants have been performed at University Hospital. Dr. Melvin did about 96 of them. He worked up to 48 hours at a stretch, averaging 18 hours a day.

Today, Dr. Melvin is director of the circulatory support devices laboratory at the University of Cincinnati Medical Center. He assists with heart transplants when needed and recovers hearts for LifeCenter. He considers us, his patients, as his closest friends. We exchange Christmas cards. We see each other at support group Christmas dinners and picnics. We are family. "There has been a lot of joy and a lot of pain," he says with mixed emotion.

The division of cardiology at University Hospital provided a lot of time and expertise to the cardiac transplant program. Dr. Peter Engel and Dr. Geetha Bhat, who in 1990 became program director of cardiac transplant (in 1997 she took a similar job running the cardiac transplant and heart failure program at Jewish Hospital of Louisville, Kentucky), put a lot of time in the program helping Dr. Melvin by evaluating potential transplant candidates and providing excellent care for them while they were on the waiting list. Much of it was their own time. "Dr. Engel was in a situation where he could do this but he could not devote nearly as much time as I needed or as he would have liked to have given," remembers Dr. Melvin.

Both Dr. Engel and Dr. Bhat were cardiologists. I still see Dr. Engel four times a year.

Dr. M. Roy First, director of transplant nephrology at University Hospital's transplant division, went all out to assist Dr. Melvin in immunosuppression.

"I didn't mind the job titles of program and surgical director," recalls Dr. Melvin. "But I did mind the work. It was a lot of work. It was equivalent to a job for two or three people. I was losing sleep and was always tired. I went from being a very young 43 to a very old 47. After the transplant, we had to do follow-up care—immunosuppression, managing other medications, and perform cardiac biopsies."

You could see during this time how much Dr. Melvin had aged. The job was taking its toll not only on him but on his family as well.

The larger heart transplant programs, and there are 141 in the United States, have larger staffs than University Hospital's in Cincinnati. Pittsburgh, Stanford, the Cleveland Clinic, and Columbia-Presbyterian in New York City have two or three different heart transplant teams. There were 2,185 heart transplants performed in 1999 in the United States. University Hospital averages 15 to 25 a year.

Dr. Melvin agrees that heart transplant programs with more than one surgical team can do more transplants. But he is quick to point out that in his first full year (1986) doing heart transplants at University Hospital, "We had the busiest first year of any heart transplant program in the world. We did 33 heart transplants in 1986. We did more than the Cleveland Clinic. We did more than St. Louis and Washington University. I think Stanford and the University of Pittsburgh did more and probably the University of Utah and the University of Minnesota.

"When we (cardiac transplant) got a consult for a patient at a Greater Cincinnati hospital that was a potential transplant candidate, I had to go see them, wherever they were—St. Luke West or Bethesda North or Mercy Hospital Clermont or the Mercy Franciscan Hospitals or Miami Valley in Dayton, Ohio. I would evaluate them and if they seemed like good candidates I would beg Peter (Engel) to make time to see them or if he wasn't available I called Geetha (Bhat) or another cardiologist to give me their opinion. If they were listed, I followed them while they were on the list. I would make rounds at all the hospitals where I had patients. I'd start out at 3:30 in the morning and then come back to University where we had people waiting in the hospital there for heart transplants. At that time, both the staff and facilities at University Hospital could not handle the load since we had so many people waiting for transplants. We had a lot of very ill people in the hospital at one time."

By 1990, Dr. Melvin was ready to relinquish the cardiac transplant program. Dr. Geetha Bhat ran the program until 1996. "I wanted to concentrate on research," says Dr. Melvin. "I've always been interested in mechanical devices. It's a passion and when I talk about it (mechanical heart-assist devices) I get into my personal philosophy of life. Basically, I think that's the only reason for doing things. We're put here to do something. I strongly believe that if the Lord wanted to hammer home to somebody the importance of long-term mechanical devices, He would put him in a situation like that where you can see people like you (me) and Wink (White) and Jack (Stranko) and see how well people do when they get a new heart and also see the impact of the organ shortage. I'm convinced that's what I was meant to do."

In the months leading up to September 1990, Dr. Melvin felt several things about the cardiac transplant program were very clear to him: the cardiac transplant program was firmly established and approaching one hundred transplants; survival rates were above the national average; and University Hospital and the UC Medical Center were going to get Medicare approval. "With new leadership from cardiology eager to direct the program, there no longer seemed to be much doubt in my mind as to the program's survival, with or without me," says Dr. Melvin.

At the same time, Dr. Melvin's research into mechanical circulatory support required not only more of his time, but more intensive preparation than he would have been able to devote to it if he was still running the transplant program. "Specifically, I needed a long period of work in a center well experienced in that research, and more formal education, probably a Ph.D. in bioengineering," he says.

Finally, Dr. Melvin wanted to spend time with his family. Before giving up the transplant program, neither Sue nor his four sons had seen much of him since the latter part of 1985. "This," he says, "would likely not have changed without major reorganization."

Shortly before 1990, only two or three other heart transplant programs in the country had Medicare approval. "Getting Medicare approval was the key to the economic viability of the program," he maintains.

So Dr. Melvin turned the reins over to a new director. At about this time, the University of Cincinnati Medical Center got a new chief of cardiology, Dr. Rick Walsh, from the University of Texas. He was gung-ho about the heart transplant program. "I couldn't have asked for it to work out any better," reflects Dr. Melvin. "What I wanted to happen, happened."

Religion guides Dr. Melvin each and every day. He is a devout Christian. "You pursue your goals based upon what you feel is important," he says. "And there are reasons you feel things are important. I think even those people who are not overtly religious, whether they know it or not, their values are there because of generations past. I think there is a limited amount of time in which those prevailing values will exist unless there's a personal involvement. There is sociologic inertia that kind of works to our benefit. I don't think it's going to work to our benefit too long unless there's more widespread personal involvement. But that's more of a philosophic opinion."

When I ask if he's very religious, Dr. Melvin gets quiet and says humbly, "Yes, I am. That is the reason for doing things."

In 1991 and 1992, Dr. Melvin was a visiting professor at the University of Vienna and The Allegemeines Krankenhaus, Vienna, working with mechanical heart-assist devices. His colleagues were Dr. Ernst Wolner, a cardiac surgeon and chief of cardiac surgery at the University of Vienna, and Heinrich (Heinz) Schima, a biomedical engineer. Both then and now, Dr. Melvin's work concentrates on ways to keep the blood-contacting surfaces—the lining of the natural heart that in most people is perfectly okay—from the artificial surfaces while supplying artificial power to the damaged heart. The heart muscle is damaged and you have to get the energy supply into the body in a way that doesn't require a hole in the skin. The Novacor® and the HeartMate® are two such devices that move the walls of the existing heart so as to avoid having the blood contact the artificial surface. "These devices are going to function as well as our native endocardium, the lining of the heart," says Dr. Melvin. The Novacor® and HeartMate® have been used on more than 15 patients waiting for a heart transplant at University Hospital in Cincinnati. "Our major interest is trying to solve some of the engineering and surgical problems related to these devices," emphasizes Dr. Melvin.

Dr. Melvin has begun his dissertation research for a Ph.D. in bioengineering at Ohio State University and is collaborating with a bioengineering group at the Cleveland Clinic.

Dr. Melvin and his colleague, Dave Glos, an aerospace engineer who did his master's work in biomechanics, are looking at the mechanical characteristics of the failing heart muscle. "But there is a big gap in what we understand," cautions Dr. Melvin. "Nobody understands what happens to the heart if you push it or squeeze it in a certain way. What we care about is when it does its own squeezing because that's what it normally does. If we have to manipulate the heart, it becomes very important to find out what its physical elastic properties are in a passive state."

Through Structural Research Dynamics Corp. (SDRC), a Milford, Ohio, mechanical software firm, and Bio/Start, a Cincinnati bio-medical incubator, they have founded CardioEnergetics.

There are four devices Dr. Melvin and Glos are working on currently. Two of them are for energy transfer to be used for circulatory support. One is a transformer that carries electrical energy from outside the body to inside the body without breaking the skin. This device is patented. The second is a method of capturing a muscle from somewhere in the body and then transferring that power to drive a cardiac-assist device. "You have a lot of spare muscles in your body to generate more than enough power," says Dr. Melvin. "The limitation is that it allows you to use only one muscle.

That would do well for about 30 to 35 beats per minute, but most human hearts beat twice as fast. Also, it can't do enough work on its own. We need to find a way to connect a muscle to an artificial device—whether it's a hydraulic linkage or cable linkage—and leave the muscles where they are while transmitting the power into the chest and heart."

The third device is another very old idea involving not a transplant or an artificial heart or a pump to assist it, but having something on or around the heart to move the heart muscle and the walls of the heart. "The advantage would be not having to replace the heart's lining and the blood contacting surface," explains Dr. Melvin. "This is important because when the heart fails, it is almost always a muscle that fails. The lining of the heart, for the most part, is usually okay. There may be some damaged areas but you can remove those."

The blood-contacting surface has been a potential problem for clots and for simply wearing out. "A new device would create different pressures on both sides of the heart," maintains Dr. Melvin. "This is hard when you are just putting something around it to keep from banging up the coronary arteries, damaging the valves, and turning them wrong-side out when you're applying these pressures. You have to allow the heart to fill rather

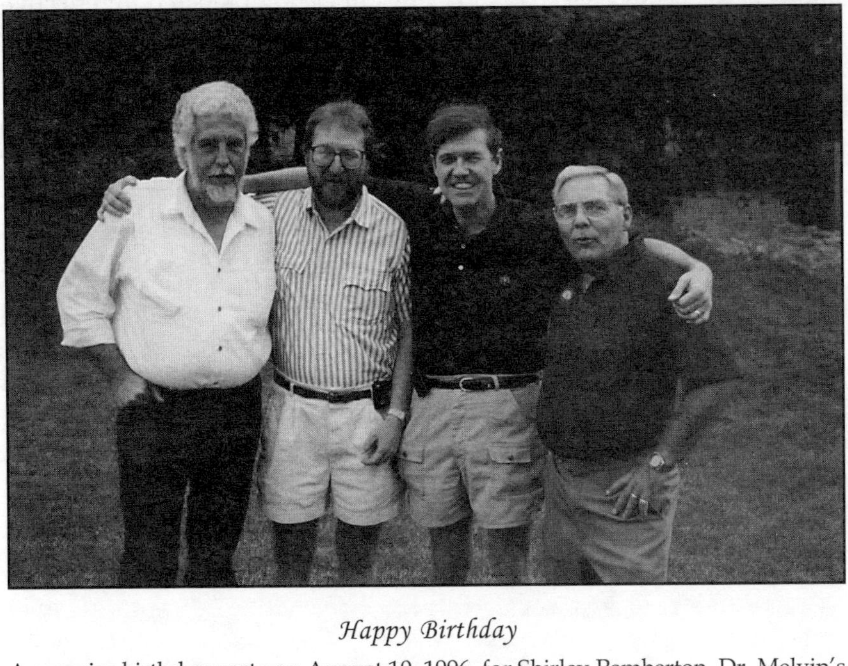

Happy Birthday

A surprise birthday party on August 10, 1996, for Shirley Pemberton, Dr. Melvin's former secretary at University Hospital's cardiac transplant program and clinic. *From left to right*: Verlin Hollon, heart recipient; Jeff Lueders; Dr. David Melvin; and Wink White, heart recipient.

Photograph © by Debbie Lueders

easily because many times a failing heart has as much trouble relaxing as it does contracting. I think we have a system that will allow that to be done."

The fourth device, a CardioClasp®, changes the shape of the heart's enlarged ventricles so that the stress on the walls can be reduced exactly as much as it can with removal of muscle. It does it by changing the shape of the heart rather than the size. The software from SDRC reduces product development time almost in half. The CardioClasp® is becoming a reality thanks to a $1 million corporate investor. Animal testing is taking place now and human testing could begin within a year.

"All these ideas have been worked on a long time without ever being totally solved," maintains Dr. Melvin. "You have to look at the number of people who need heart transplants, the number who have already had them, and the remaining problems that stand between us and a viable mechanical heart-assist device that is affordable and safe in order to help make a contribution. Between myself and other researchers who have experienced and learned the problems of cardiac transplantation, I think the chances are pretty good we'll make a contribution sometime in the next 15 years." Dr. Melvin is very proud of the cardiac transplant program at University Hospital that he helped found. He is equally proud of his current research and believes he and his laboratory are sufficiently prepared for effective research that is compatible with more active clinical work and trials.

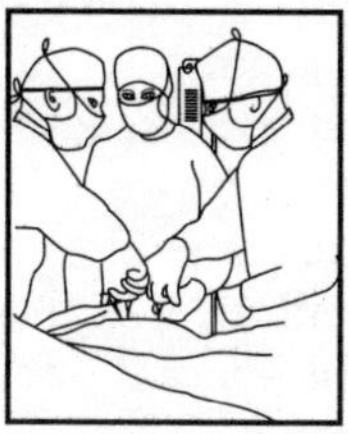

4

Faith

To learn the true meaning of faith, you need only reach for your Bible and read the Book of Job. I am not the most religious man, but I do try to attend church regularly. I did not make it through my heart transplant without the prayers of friends, neighbors, and co-workers. At times my faith wavered and I did not attend church. Blaming God for my health problems was easy. But it was not the answer. The answer lay in faith and prayer.

When Jesus called his disciples in the Book of Matthew, he gave them authority over unclean spirits, to cast them out, and to heal every disease and every infirmity. Peter and Andrew, brothers who were fisherman, were made "fishers of men." All 12 of the disciples gave away everything they owned and had worked for to follow Jesus because they had faith.

In Matthew 19:16–22, we learn why it is hard for a rich man to enter the kingdom of heaven. And behold, one came to him saying, "Teacher, what good deed must I do, to have eternal life?" And he (Jesus) said to him, "Why do you ask me about what is good? One there is who is good. If you would enter life, keep the commandments." He said to him, "Which?" And Jesus said, "You shall not kill, You shall not commit adultery, You shall not steal, You shall not bear false witness, Honor your mother and father, and You shall love your neighbor as yourself." The young man said to him, "All these I have observed; what do I still lack?" Jesus said to him, "If you would be perfect, go, sell what you possess and give it to the poor, and you will have treasure in heaven; and come follow me." When the young man heard this he went away sorrowful; for he had great possessions.

The Reverend Billy Graham says that faith is a fact and that you must disregard your feelings. Feeling does not save you, and you may or may not feel the Spirit. Accept Him (Jesus) by faith as a fact. He lives within you right now to help you live the Christian life. He is living in you so that you can live a happy, victorious, radiant, Christ-honoring life.

While I was waiting for my heart transplant, I tried to accept the wait as best I could. My name was placed on a list of people nationwide. The

United States is divided into regions for organ allocation. I was in the Ohio, Indiana, and Michigan region. University Hospital in Cincinnati, a transplant center, was part of a computerized national network of organ identification and sharing. There were approximately 18,500 people in the United States in February 1989 waiting for an organ transplant when I went on the list. UNOS, based in Richmond, Virginia, oversees organ allocation according to national organ sharing policies established by the Organ Procurement and Transplantation Network. The policies are approved by the U.S. Department of Human Services. UNOS, operating on a local, regional, and national basis, is under contract with the federal government. UNOS also provides research and scientific data to its members and the general public. Its members include 61 organ procurement organizations (OPOs), 261 transplant centers and 854 transplant programs around the country, and tissue typing laboratories.

The goals I set for myself revolved around staying alive long enough to receive the transplant. Dr. Melvin and his staff at the cardiac transplant program of University Hospital indicated I had a 50/50 chance of making it through 1989. In essence, it sounded like I had six months to live. I had to learn to deal with this sobering news. I had to deal with potentially stressful situations in a constructive manner. I tried to maintain my health by eating a well-balanced low-fat diet and exercising moderately, though just walking from room to room tired me, as did climbing the shortest flight of stairs.

My suitcase remained packed and sitting in the hallway so I could quickly leave for the hospital as soon as a new heart was available. I tried to get on with my life while waiting. I even took several literature courses from the University of Cincinnati to take my mind off the wait and my worsening condition.

Throughout the wait, there was a considerable amount of stress to deal with. I suppose deep down, even though I prayed constantly for a new heart, I was scared. I was not scared of dying, for I had come to accept that as a definite possibility. I had some fear of the unknown—how I would do after transplant, how quickly I could return to work, how I would feel with someone else's heart. Through a support group called Change of Heart, the social worker, Kathy Gosney, and the transplant coordinator, Julie Collins, I was able to channel my energies into creative, constructive, and worthwhile activities as I waited. By talking to my minister, The Reverend Calvin Klumb at Pilgrim United Church of Christ (in Bridgetown on Cincinnati's west side) where I attend, a psychologist and my friends, I was able to put my concerns in perspective while at the same time relieving stress and frustration.

I would lie awake at night, partly because I had trouble breathing and partly because I could not sleep, and just listen to the faint beat of my weak heart. Soon, I prayed, a new and stronger heart would beat in its place. I had to keep this last hope alive. I had to have faith. I guess I did, whether I worshipped in church on Sunday or not. God was with me wherever I went. I read and re-read "Footprints in the Sand." I read the Bible. I even took a two-year Bible-study course called Kerygma.

During the year and a half I was off work, and before I even went on the waiting list for a heart at University Hospital, I tried to keep my body, mind, and spirit as one (John 17:21). It was hard. My faith was severely tested. It is easy to have a lot of faith when things are going well in your life. But throw people a curve like a catastrophic illness and not even the most dedicated and persuasive member of the clergy can convince you that it is not God's will to make you suffer. I like to call this phase the "Why me, God?" syndrome. I'm sure it is a universal feeling of all those who have or are suffering from catastrophic illnesses. I even stopped going to church for a while and lost faith. I gave up on God. But God never gave up on me. I know that now because he kept me alive long enough to have my heart transplant.

Because of my mom and grandma's strong faith, Rev. Calvin Klumb, my best friend, and his wife, Dan and Renae Stenger, and many other church friends, I came to realize that God allowed this heart disease to happen to me. So instead of being angry and jealous of my friends and neighbors who all had good health, I began to pray and have faith in God. My wife, Debbie, always tries to tell me not to be envious of others because of their wealth, status, or material things they have, but to be thankful for all the good things in life we have – good jobs, a nice home, and most of all, love.

Though death crossed my mind, I was neither afraid nor worried about it. I am a heart transplant recipient now and I know I'm eventually going to die. But everybody dies. Every person who comes into this world dies.

I was reading an interesting article in The Reverend Billy Graham's magazine, *Decision* (October 1996). Dr. David L. Stevens, executive director for the Christian Medical and Dental Society in Bristol, Tennessee, wrote the article, "When You Die, What Will Happen to You?" He has been a missionary doctor in Kenya, Russia, Somalia, and the Sudan. Death is prevalent in these countries because of a lack of medical care and primitive conditions. But Stevens found that all people, no matter what culture, seem preoccupied with death. "Many traditional African tribal dances, for example, deal with themes of death, spirits, and returning ancestors," he says. "Many Eastern religious practices include the worship of dead relatives. The alarming rise of occultism and spiritism in Western countries has spread a fascination with contacting the dead through psychic means. The teachings of the New Age movement have emphasized notions such as reincarnation."

Stevens identified the things about death that concern people.

Death implies judgment: "It is appointed for men to die once and after this judgment comes" (Hebrews 9:27).

Death testifies to the consequence of sin: "Through one man sin entered into the world, and death through sin, and so death spread to all men because all sinned" (Romans 5:12).

Death denies our independence: "No man has authority to retain the spirit, or authority over the day of death; there is no discharge from war, nor will wickedness deliver those who are given to it" (Ecclesiastes 8:8).

Death ends speculation: "Yea, he shall see that even the wise die, the fool and the stupid alike must perish" (Psalm 49:10).

Like others facing catastrophic illnesses, I did not know what to expect or how to feel about facing death. And I came very, very close to death. Stevens maintains that death is the result of man's choice, not God's plan: "From the tree of the knowledge of good and evil you shall not eat, for in the day that you eat from it you shall surely die" (Genesis 2:17).

And says Stevens, God still offers us a choice between life and death: "I call heaven and earth to witness against you today, that I have set before you life and death, the blessing and the curse. So choose life in order that you may live, you and your descendants" (Deuteronomy 30:19).

I chose life. Stevens says we can rest assured that we have eternal life if we believe in and receive Jesus Christ: "God has given us eternal life, and this life is in His Son. He who has the Son has the life; he who does not have the Son of God does not have the life" (1 John 5:11–12).

Stevens sums up the article by concluding, "God has entrusted to us the answers to life's most pressing questions. He has given us his Word that we can not only have eternal life ourselves, but we can also lead others to new life in Christ."

It is inevitable that I will die; everyone dies. The only lasting impact I can make on the lives of my wife, Debbie, my mom, Adele, my mother-in-law, Alma, along with other family, friends, and colleagues, is to show them the way that leads from death to life.

* * * * *

I know my heart transplant was a gift from God. It was a miracle. When my mom was hospitalized in February 1985 for a mastectomy for breast cancer, I thought I was going to lose her. I was scared and frightened. But I prayed, along with my grandma and all our friends in the neighborhood and at church. Mom came through with flying colors. She did not even need any radiation or chemotherapy treatments. It is September 2000, and she has been cancer-free for 15 years. I thank God for that every night, along with a prayer for Debbie, Brandon, and his family, and the rest of our families. But my faith is tested every day. On December 4, 1996, Mom told me she thought she felt a lump in her other breast. Right away, anger set in instead of faith. I told God if this proved to be cancer, I would never set foot in church again. I would pledge no money. Several days later she saw her family doctor and had her yearly mammogram. Everything was normal. I apologized again to God for my lack of faith. I'm sure my faith will be tested again and again. Maybe next time I will have more faith. I will try.

On January 9, 1997, Mom had a knee replacement at Mercy Franciscan Hospital-Western Hills Campus, in Cincinnati. Things went very well. She was in the hospital 12 days. When she came home, a six-week rehabilitation program began. It went remarkably well. By the beginning of March, she was driving and able to walk very well without pain. I had faith from the beginning. That made all the difference in the world. Mom is 79.

While Mom was hospitalized 15 years ago in 1985, one of her church friends, Martha Fowler, gave her a prayer book. It is called *Beside Still Waters*. It is comprised of prayers, poems, and inspirational thoughts. When Mom and I both moved, in 1995 and 1996, somehow I ended up with the book. She had used it a lot for devotions at her Ladies Guild meetings. I opened the book as I was starting to write this chapter, looking for a prayer or thought about losing your faith and then regaining it. I did not find one. What I did find was a poem/prayer called "Today."

> *My life is a gift of God, given not in years, but a day at a time. Today is the day the Lord has made for me, and He planned it to be the most important day of my life.*
>
> *Yesterday is gone, never to return. I must not worry about it, but leave it in the hands of God. Tomorrow and all that it holds is God's secret and its coming is not assured. Only today is mine. Each day, arranged by God with infinite wisdom and goodness is His gift, His act of love for me. In thanksgiving I will offer Him every day the gift of myself – my prayers, works, joys and sufferings.*
>
> *Dear Lord, receive it graciously.*

I know now that this is exactly how I should feel each day. And I will reread this beautiful poem every time I forget just how blessed I am. I have only to look at the beauty of my surroundings—the pale blue sky and snow white clouds that resemble cotton balls; the green fertile grass and fields of flowers and trees; the autumn colors; the drifting snow in winter; a spring shower; a clear summer night with a harvest moon—to know that only God could have made all these. He watches over us all.

Perhaps my heart transplant has brought me closer to God and strengthened my faith. I tend to get mad when my computer isn't working right or something goes wrong at the office or I lose in basketball. And I blame God! Sternly and sometimes with anger, Debbie chastises me for this. She is right. I'm sure my faith will still waver at times. But I know God loves me. I pray every day. I know God is with me with every breath I take, with every basket I shoot on the court, with every step I walk or run. I gave up on God before the heart transplant. God never gave up on me. I received a second chance at life. I am making the most of this second chance. God lives within me. I must deal with life's challenges.

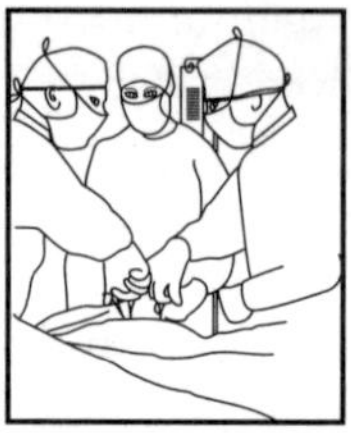

5

Soul mates

Grow old along with me!
The best is yet to be,
The last of life, for which the first was made:
Our times are in His hand
Who saith, 'A whole I planned,
Youth shows but half; trust God: see all, nor be afraid!'

—"Rabbi ben Ezra," by Robert Browning,
written for his wife, Elizabeth Barrett Browning

Webster's defines soul mate as a person temperamentally suited to another. I found my soul mate six years ago in 1994. She was almost like the girl next door. The only trouble was I did not know she lived close by me for almost 20 years.

Sometimes you find love when you least expect it. That is the way it was with me. I was 39 and resigned myself to the fact I would probably be a bachelor the rest of my life.

I do not know too much about that quest to find your soul mate, but I had my own transforming journey that author Richard Bach wrote about in *One,* as he magically discovered love and joy and a sense of freedom. Debbie and I had a love at first sight relationship. Our courtship was brief. When you finish each other's thoughts and sentences, and know what you both want out of life, the rest comes pretty naturally.

More than anything else, Debbie has taught me to find the good in everyone and everything. She does not think that money is the measure of a man. She has taught me to be thankful for the good things in life we have—good health and a nice home and family—not to be envious of what others have. Her faith in God is steadfast. I would like to think my faith is too.

When you find your soul mate, as I have, the world is a better place. It is real nice waking up next to someone every morning. Debbie exalts in my triumphs and picks me up when I am down. She seldom raises her voice or gets angry, even when I am at fault. This is not to say we see eye to eye on everything. We were married relatively late in our lives and are very set in our ways. As I am fond of saying, "She hasn't begun to think like a Lueders quite as quickly as I'd like."

Soul mates share everything: hopes, dreams, tomorrows, todays, yesterdays. Debbie and I often think if we had only met 20 years ago, we could have had children and be looking forward to grandchildren. But we are happy we just found each other.

I love everything about Debbie. I love her hair. I love the way she walks. I love the way she looks in sweatpants and shorts. I love looking at her when she is asleep. I love holding her at night. I love touching her. I love making love to her. I love how she dresses. I love her cooking and baking.

Though she was born in Kentucky, Debbie grew up in Dayton, Ohio, where she says she was always sort of a shy kid who preferred to read or sew than play outside. "When I was about five or six, my parents sent me to dance classes where I learned the fine art of ballet, toe, and tap dancing for about six years. Every year we'd have a recital and we had the prettiest costumes of satins, silks, and sequins. Those costumes are all packed away somewhere in a box in my mother's house. One of my favorite costumes my grandmother made me was a little white satin outfit with puff sleeves with green shimmery shamrocks all over with an emerald green weskit that laced up the front and then I had glittery silver tap shoes with matching green satin ribbons. I did some form of an Irish jig that year. Some years I had several numbers, some tap and some ballet or toe. It was a fun experience. I can still remember all the rehearsals and the piano player pounding out those tunes we danced to. Funny how little things like that stick in your mind. Anyway, by the time I was about 12, my parents bought a new spinet piano and by that time I was a little tired of dancing lessons, so I quit that and started piano lessons. I really enjoyed the piano and even took a class in college, where as a senior, my music professor tried to get me to change my major from textiles and design to music—which I didn't do, much to my parents' relief. I also played softball in the eighth grade and graduated from Dayton's Fairview High School, the same school that baseball Hall of Famer Mike Schmidt graduated from several years earlier."

Debbie's dad, Bill Pritchett, was a retired lieutenant colonel in the Army Reserves. He was a veteran of World War II and the Korean War, earning medals like the Purple Heart, and the Silver and Bronze Star. He was in a battle called the Punch Bowl that included Heartbreak Ridge and Bloody Ridge under the direction of Colonel Boatwright. "Dad never talked much about the war though," says Debbie, "except to mention that his feet had been frostbitten one winter during the war."

Her dad's career began at Globe Industries in Dayton where he worked for 15 years in the quality control department. The company was bought out by giant TRW and he lost his job in the reorganization. "By that time, I was just starting college at Eastern Kentucky University in Richmond," remembers Debbie. "So after job hunting in Dayton and finding no suitable jobs, he contacted a friend in Cincinnati who ran an employment agency who gave him a few leads on jobs in Cincinnati. After several interviews he was hired by the 3M Company as their quality assurance manager.

"Meanwhile, my mom, Alma, had been working in Dayton at the Kissell Company, a mortgage banking company, since I had started grade school. She was lucky enough to transfer to their Cincinnati branch where she eventually became office manager. She was with Kissell for 33 years. Even though she's retired now, her knowledge of mortgage banking has come in handy on numerous occasions—when we got married and purchased a condo and more recently when we refinanced the condo. She and my grandmother were always there for me and were invaluable in helping me through two back surgeries. I'm also very proud of her for quitting smoking recently after smoking one pack a day for almost 50 years. That really takes a lot of will power."

While her mom and dad both worked, Debbie's grandmother, Christine Combs, took care of her when she was growing up. "She lived with Mom until she died of pneumonia on February 2, 1999, at the age of 90. I was probably five or six years old when she came to live with us," says Debbie. "Since we were little tykes, my cousins and I have always called her Nan, but when she was out in the working world her nickname was 'Teen.' She grew up on a farm where all the kids were expected to do their chores. She could tell stories about riding her horse to the little one room schoolhouse in Owsley County, Kentucky. Her dad was a schoolteacher and her mom ran the farm. Nan was a wonderful cook who cooked most everything from scratch, with no recipe of course. I learned the basics of cooking and sewing at her elbow. Particularly in sewing she always taught me that if you don't do something the right way, then you pick it out and start all over until you get it right. The end result of that teaching is that I won several ribbons from local fairs and craft contests for my counted cross-stitch pictures, most of which were made for special people and were given away. She made beautiful quilts in her day and I had asked her to show me the 'how-to's' of quilting. I have my first project pieced and started the quilting, but still don't have it finished yet.

"Jeff likes to tell everyone that since he married me, he's related to former New York Yankee and Baseball Hall of Famer, Earle Combs, who played with Babe Ruth and Lou Gehrig. Actually we're sort of distantly related. My grandfather, Chester Combs, and Earle Combs had the same great-great-great-grandfather, Mason Combs (1714–1785). I do like to dabble in genealogy when I have time. Mom's line of Roses, Stewarts, Reynolds,

Moores, Bowmans, and Combs were early pioneers to central Kentucky, especially in Owsley County. Several ancestors were supposedly traced back to England and Germany in the 1600s. There are some interesting stories in all that family history—tales of family divisions during the Civil War, Revolutionary War heroes, and ancestors that emigrated to America on ships like the *Marigold* and the *Francis and John* in the early 1600s.

"We don't have much family left these days. Dad passed away in 1985 from pancreatic cancer when I was 35. Jeff's dad died in 1977 from two massive heart attacks. Jeff was 22. We both miss our dads and when we were married we added a little note to the back of our programs that said a *special word of thanks to our dads who we're sure are smiling down on us today as we're thinking of them.*

"I wrote in my diary that my wedding day was the happiest day of my life, and I truly meant it. That's one thing about marrying when you're older, you have a lot more friends to share with and celebrate with on your wedding day. I visited with old high school and college friends like Roxie Gates and Marian Allen who I hadn't seen in 25 years and our remaining aunts, uncles, and cousins from Oregon and Georgia, played a big part in the wedding too. My cousin Kathy Ritter, several years younger than I, was one of my bridesmaids and caught my bouquet and now she's a married lady! Never say never as they say. My college roommate, Caryn Helms, who I graduated with 28 years ago, was a bridesmaid, and traveled from eastern Kentucky. My friend Gilda Young, who I had worked with in the surgical resident office at the University of Cincinnati College of Medicine for about five years, was my matron of honor. She is a sweet, Christian lady who had gotten married for the first time only several years before me and always extolled the joys of married life and said she would have to 'find me a man.' Now that we're married, Jeff and I always are on the lookout for any potential mates for our single friends. We just want everyone to be as happy as we are.

"It still amazes me to this day what close proximity Jeff and I were to each other, to never have known one another. His church was right around the corner from mine. His mom's house and my mom's house were in the same neighborhood. We even had some of the same friends, sort of. I worked with Ann Demmy, a nurse and transplant coordinator for the kidney/pancreas patients. Her husband, John, knew Jeff very well from the YMCA and their work on various committees together. They live close by and it's fun to get together with them as a couple now."

Debbie has an amusing anecdote about Dr. Melvin, who performed my heart transplant in 1989. "The year Jeff had his transplant, I was working in the resident office which was just around the corner from the cardiothoracic division and Dr. Melvin's office. We kept a big candy jar in our office for the residents since they often would miss meals working as they did, and Dr. Melvin stopped in for a piece of candy every now and then. One day, during the Christmas season, he came by with a big bag of M & M's to replenish our supply. How nice he is, I thought. I think I almost bumped into him a couple of times, coming around the corner, because he was always moving so fast and both of us weren't always looking where we were going. I always wondered if he was running after a heart when I saw him speed by. Dr. Melvin was another person that seemed really surprised but very pleased that I was marrying a patient of his."

* * * * *

On Valentine's Day 1997, I sent Debbie flowers with a vase and a cuddly bear. We also went to dinner. She got me candy in a mug with a helium heart balloon that said, "Wild Thing, You Make My Heart Sing!" She also got me a Dan Fogelberg CD. She wanted to get me a pair of boxer shorts with a heart on each cheek and a smiley face in front, but she couldn't find which store advertised them. We got each other very nice Valentine cards.

We never talk politics because I believe we are on opposite ends of the political spectrum. She still won't tell me whom she voted for in 1996 for president. And it doesn't bother me in the least. Well, it does, but there is not much I can do about it.

With my new heart, I have a new beginning. Though my end may come faster than I hope, I live a quality life with someone I love very much and who loves me. Who knows, with technology rapidly advancing, maybe an artificial heart is in my future. I certainly do not discount this possibility.

What I do know is that it is very nice to have someone to wake up to each morning. The day has more meaning. Nights are not lonely. More than anything else, Debbie and I live on love. We always will. It's nice to know you'll spend the rest of your life with someone you love and admire. We see through each other's faults. She helps me when I'm feeling down and I hope I do the same with her. Her kindness and understanding is something I treasure. And so do many, many others, among them doctors and nurses. Her love is unconditional.

Debbie never says a swear word. Well, it's so seldom that you could say never. Unfortunately, my vocabulary is not as good as hers. I don't pride myself on this. And I do try to watch myself, especially when we have company.

It is hard to explain how you can know someone for only a few years and feel like you have known him or her for a lifetime.

If I feel I'm getting depressed, Debbie is always there to pick me up. Sometimes she understands why I am depressed. At other times, she does not. Still, her love and affection are great comfort.

Having had a heart transplant, I realize that daily immunosuppressive medications, laboratory work, and other necessary follow-up care are vital for my existence. I accept this as my destiny, for my life has already been extended beyond what I believed possible 12 years ago. I thank God daily for my donor and donor family.

Debbie describes our romance like this:

Once upon a time there was a young lad named Jeffrey and a young lass named Deborah. Now Deborah was the secretary for not only two transplant surgeons/professors but also the organ procurement center, Ohio Valley Organ Procurement (OVOP, now LifeCenter). Lo and behold, one day this young man came to work for OVOP. He had received a heart transplant several years ago, so he was able to spread the word, not only in public education but in public relations as well. And the word was good. He became stronger and healthier than he had ever been. He could play basketball and racquetball with 'normal' people, and win. How he loved to play basketball.

Well this young woman was intrigued by this young man and his amazing progress. She learned that he lived in her neighborhood and that he liked to walk every day for his heart's sake. Since she also had to walk every day due to two back surgeries, she had developed some cassette tapes with 'music to walk to.' When it came time for the young man's birthday in January 1994, she gift wrapped a tape and gave it to him, saying that perhaps they could go walking together sometime since they lived so close.

Well, lo and behold, in April 1994 the young lad asked the young lass for a date at Playhouse in the Park, a regional theatre in Cincinnati. And behold, they were smitten with one another. And when they kissed, their lips tingled and they got all weak in the knees. They would stare deep into one another's eyes and become lost in love. After several dates the young man declared that he was "crazy in love" and in turn the young woman said she too was falling in love.

Soon after that the couple started talking about marriage in more serious terms. Would it be possible for two people of middle age who had never married and who had been so dependent on their families during their health crises to become an independent couple on their own? We decided, 'YES! It could be done!'

An engagement ring was purchased and the wedding date was set for May 20, 1995. The Change of Heart support group for heart transplant recipients was thrilled with the news and embraced the couple with hearty congratulations. Their friends were ecstatic. Their families were dumbfounded at first, not believing how fast things were moving.

And so the young man who had appeared on TV, been quoted in newspapers, and been heard on the radio promoting the cause of organ and tissue donation was finally ready to settle down.

So, for a whole year they planned every detail of their wedding. And the day finally arrived. ♥ And they smiled at each other. ♥♥ And they said, 'I do!' ♥♥♥ They kissed. ♥♥♥♥ And they lived happily ever after…♥♥♥♥♥(A very long time in fairy tale years!)

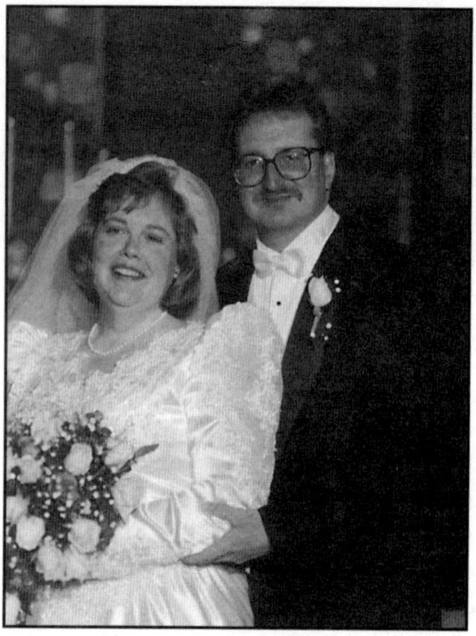

Tying the Knot

Debbie and Jeff Lueders at their wedding, May 20, 1995

Photograph © by Lancaster Photography

Which only goes to show you that prayers and dreams can come true even in real life when you trust in the Lord.

– Debbie Pritchett
May 1995

Debbie gave this to me on our second anniversary. She wrote it when we were sending our wedding invitations. Everyone kept asking her where, how, when we had met and she considered just passing this out, but instead put it in her album of wedding mementos until she shared it with me. Actually, she said it was a lot of fun telling everyone about our engagement and wedding. The other fun thing was opening all the wedding presents. She'd save all the gifts that arrived through the week and then on the weekend my mom and I would join Debbie, her mom, and grandma as we opened all the gifts. I told her, "It's just like Christmas!"

What she didn't mention was the story about the cinnamon rolls. I had the audacity to walk into her office a year or so before we even started to date, saying, "I hear you bake things for people's birthdays. My birthday is January 21 and I know you bake a mean cinnamon roll." I asked her to bake me some cinnamon rolls when I hardly knew her in 1992. I was very forward, but it was true about her excellent baking skills. She told me afterwards she asked Tom Craycraft, a transplant coordinator for OVOP (LifeCenter's former acronym), "Who is that guy?" She thought I was nervy. Needless to say her fairy tale is very special. She keeps a diary too. I told her this was just what I needed for this chapter. I'm pretty new at this romance thing, but sometimes just knowing you are loved and needed is enough. And knowing you can love in return.

The one thing all of us need in this life is unconditional love. It must be real love. It must be from the heart. Mine was love at first sight. To love and be loved is to be nurtured in mind, body, and spirit. Being loved means we can give love in return and make the world a little better place in which to live. God has a plan for all of us. He loves us for who we are and for who we can become. It is never too late to fall in love.

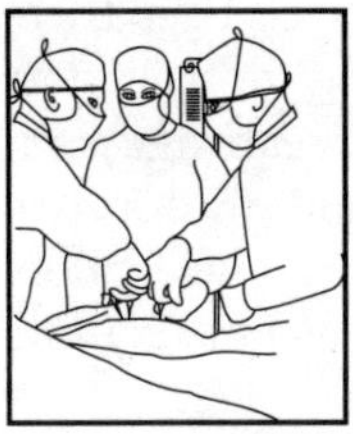

6

Friends

When I was a senior in high school, caught up in a varsity sport and eagerly awaiting college, our English class read a short novel by Richard Bach. *Jonathan Livingston Seagull* taught me many lessons about life. It was a simple story, really. A seagull trying to find the meaning of kindness and love and what being friends really meant. Jonathan was an outcast in a world where other seagulls had already found a place in life. Jonathan searched a lifetime to find true happiness and love. And all the time it was right there in his generous heart.

To me, that's what being a friend is all about. Having someone you trust and who trusts you. Someone who is a good listener. Friendship is forged on honesty, truthfulness, and wisdom. When you're in trouble, friends drop their plans to offer comfort and solace. They share in your triumphs and feel sad when things don't work out. They encourage dreams and offer advice.

Over the years, I have been blessed with great friends. A few I have known practically all my life. Through the Gamble-Nippert YMCA I have made friends with people who are like my second family. When I was close to death, they helped me hang on, through prayer, kind deeds and positive actions. Art McCue, until his death on December 22, 1999, Charlie Warner, Dave Saunders, Wilbur Franke, Mike Frith, Joe Tucker, and many more.

A few of my friends and I completed grade school, junior high, and high school together. Many I don't see or hear from often, but just thinking about them and the memories we shared, keep them vivid in my mind.

Other friends I know on a professional basis. Jim Wilson, an English professor at the University of Cincinnati, encouraged me to write this book. I met Randy McNutt, a *Cincinnati Enquirer* reporter for more than 25 years, in graduate school in 1989. We became friends immediately.

Every Tuesday night from late March until October, I play basketball outdoors at Jim and Ann Metz's. I've known Jim since the 1970s when we met at the local YMCA. Two-on-two, three-on-three, we play until it gets dark. Terry Metz, Gene Metz, Dave Simpson, Paul Meyer, and Jerry Mellencamp are some of the guys I play with.

Friends at church are very special. Debbie and I now attend both Bridgetown Church of Christ and Pilgrim United Church of Christ, my church. I have been a member there all my life and my mom has been there for more than 50 years. The friends we have there, including the ministers like Cal Klumb and Glen Halbe (both of whom left several years ago) and Bob Girard, have seen me through some very bleak times and my survival is due in large part to the thoughts and prayers of this giving congregation. I have served three board terms at Pilgrim—one on the Board of Lay Life and Work and two on the Board of Stewards.

Best friends become old friends. In the winter of 1977, I met someone I could love like a brother. His name is Dan Stenger. He comes from a hardworking family from Cleves, Ohio. He has three younger brothers, Brian, Mark and Vince, an older sister, Diane, and a younger sister, Debbie.

On October 12, 1985, Dan married Renae Schnitzler. I was his best man. I was also very, very sick at the time. "At first you didn't know what was wrong," remembers Dan. "You were pretty down about it when the doctors discovered it was your heart. I didn't know what to think. When they found out it was a heart problem, I was pretty scared. I didn't know what to do to help you either. There were times when you couldn't even get out of bed."

Two of Dan's uncles had kidney transplants at University Hospital. Jim Stenger had his transplant in 1981 and lived seven years. He died of cancer. He was also one of the first kidney transplant recipients to undergo bypass surgery at University Hospital. Tom Stenger, a partner in a Cincinnati general contracting firm, had his kidney transplant in 1984 and has resumed his normal workload and family life.

After my heart transplant, Dan says he "was amazed" at my quick recovery. "You were so ill before the transplant and you had very little energy. And then I went in to see you the day after the surgery and you were perked up in bed. You had this major cut in your chest but you looked 100 percent better. It was amazing. Renae and I felt better too.

"I admired your determination to get back in the workforce and your going back to school. Then you met someone. Renae and I felt like we were parents. Your romance with Debbie went so fast. We're both so happy for you.

"Through your whole ordeal, I remember not knowing how to support you. There's no way for someone who is not experiencing a catastrophic illness can really understand all you were going through."

Dan and Renae exemplify the true meaning of friends. Sometimes it's hard to come right out and say you love someone. But I love Dan and Renae.

Vince, Dan's brother, lives near the University of Cincinnati where he's working on a graduate engineering degree. Even though I seldom see him we send e-mail to one another, talk occasionally on the telephone, and get together.

When I got married and my mom sold her house, we moved away from neighbors we had known more than 30 years—dear friends like Joe Gramaglia whose wife, Helen, died on November 11, 1997. Helen and my mom went to high school together. Our next-door neighbors for 18 years, Dennis and Sharon McManus, and Kelly, Tracy and Kevin, were almost like family. Dennis was in our wedding. Now we seem miles apart though we live less than a mile from each other.

I know these friends will be friends for life.

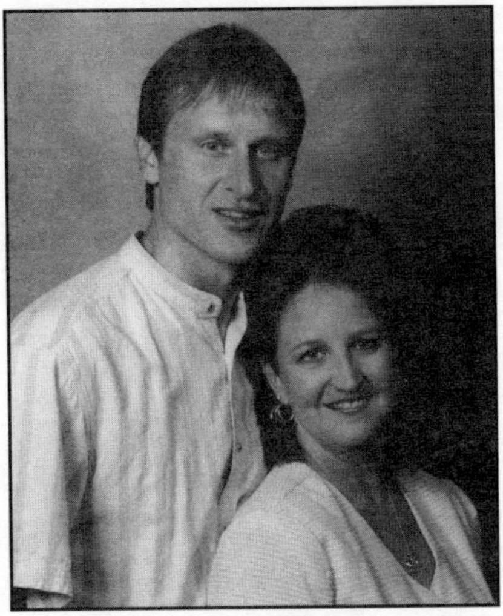

Friends Forever

Best friends, Dan and Renae Stenger

Photograph © by American School Picture

Section II

Donor Family Stories

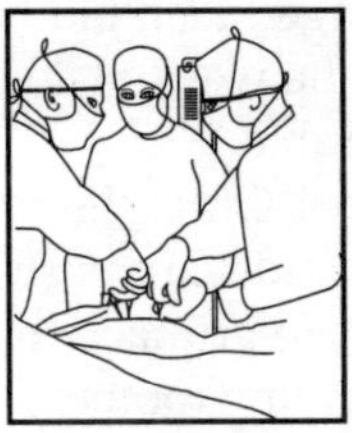

7

Brandon Burress: an athlete with a future

As a heart transplant recipient, I thank God each day, along with the transplant team, my supportive family, and friends. There is also a daily prayer for the donor I never knew or met, and the donor family. My family, especially my wife, Debbie, and I have a warm feeling inside knowing that because of a donor family's love, kindness, and courage, I have not only been renewed physically, but also enriched by one family's humanity to another.

Donor families are very special. In times of extreme anguish and unbearable pain, their courage and fortitude supersede their grief, allowing them to help others live. Often times they know their loved one's wishes about donation because they have discussed them as a family. They can make a decision to comply with their loved one's wishes when approached by transplant coordinators and hospital healthcare professionals involved in the request process. It is a decision that would make their loved ones proud. Caring and sensitive healthcare professionals help these individuals make the toughest decision of their lives. For donor families, it is the ultimate sacrifice.

* * * * *

In the early summer of 1989, I was languishing on the waiting list of the cardiac transplant program at University Hospital in Cincinnati. I was fast approaching six months on the list. Without a heart transplant, I would have died. At the same time, in Blanchester, Ohio, east of Cincinnati, a young man was hard at work toning his mind, body, and spirit for the upcoming football season at Blanchester High School. That summer, he began conditioning in the weight room of the high school. Every day he rode his bike eight miles one way to the high school. At six feet and 185 pounds, he was as dedicated as they come. In a few short months, after summer vacation, he would be a freshman at Blanchester High School. His name was Brandon Burress. He was 15 years old.

"Brandon was a good kid growing up," says his mother, Sheree Starr. When Debbie, my fiance at the time (April 23, 1995), and I visited with her and her family in her Blanchester, Ohio, home, they all spoke enthusiastically about Brandon. "I didn't have any problems with him. He and his friends stayed away from drugs and alcohol. He got on edge like all kids do. But basically I did not have to worry about him when he was outside playing. I did not have to worry about him getting into trouble."

His maternal grandmother, Norma Jean Rieke, of Cleves, Ohio, shows me a picture of Brandon at eight, when he was in the third grade. His curly blond hair stands out as he poses in his football uniform. He grimaces in the photo. "He told us you had to look tough if you were playing football," remembers Norma fondly.

At 11, he attended Blanchester Middle School. His mom and grandma say he always liked school. By the time he was 15, Brandon began to make some important decisions about his life. Growing up without a father—James Burress left Brandon and Sheree when Brandon was an infant—he knew he was now the man of the family, watching over his mom and his younger sister and brother. He talked about going to college, becoming a police officer, or maybe joining the Air Force.

At 15, he was more mature than some kids much older. He still liked school. He had a girlfriend, or as his mom put it, "There was one particular girl he liked. They saw each other at school but that was about it. There were a lot of girls who liked him. They used to drive up and down our road looking for him. Not having a telephone or a car left Brandon stuck at the house."

On the afternoon of June 26, 1989, Brandon's hopes and dreams for the future ended. He and his friend David Hughes, a Blanchester Junior High football player, were riding their bikes back from Blanchester. They had gone to Blanchester High School for weight training but found the weight room locked. Varsity coach at that time was Bob Braman. He said weight training was from 6–8 P.M. Brandon and David rode their bikes into Blanchester, stopping at a drugstore to buy batteries for their remote cars and blank cassette tapes. Brandon also bought a bottle of hair coloring or dye at a sundry store. Then, they headed home. It is unclear whether they planned to return to the high school at 6 P.M. At 4:25 P.M., a car driven by Rick Fenner hit Brandon. Fenner, who's now about 29, was a Blanchester High School graduate, and a former quarterback, basketball and baseball player who began attending Miami University in the fall of 1989. The accident happened on Clermont County Road, State Route 133, north of Taylor Road in Wayne Township. It was 92 degrees that Monday, hot, humid and hazy. The sun was out very little. The asphalt road was straight and level. Fenner's car was a 1984 white, two-door Chevrolet Cavalier, Ohio license 753 TAB. Brandon was riding a Kent Diplomat 3000 10-speed bicycle. Fenner said he was going the speed limit, 55 mph. Brandon was hit and thrown from his bike. David, scared by the honking of Fenner's horn, ended up in a ditch on the right side of the road. David was not hurt and managed to get to Sheree's but no one was home and she did not have a telephone. Goshen, Wayne, and Harlan Township rescue squads, EMTs, and paramedics responded to the accident. The Ohio State Highway Patrol handled the accident investigation and report. Brandon suffered a severe closed head injury, anoxic brain damage, scapula fracture, and multiple abrasions.

EMT Andy Mitten of the Harlan Township Fire Department recalls he was on the scene and it was Harlan Township's task to set up a landing zone for Air Care. "I remember driving up to the scene and I remember the vehicles and the people. I was not one of the first on the scene. I saw the car, the caved in windshield, and the bicycle. I know they were doing cardiopulmonary resuscitation (CPR) on him at the time. I had my camcorder with me. I don't know why, but I did not have my department vehicle. I had our red family van. I remember walking around videotaping the car and the bicycle. While they were working on him I videotaped some of when they took him over to the helicopter and took off. Wayne Township was already there and I remember Brandon was lying on the highway. He was flown by University Hospital's Air Care helicopter to the hospital's trauma unit."

There was a little farmhouse on State Route 133 called Green Towers. "He (Rick Fenner) used their telephone to call home," says Sheree.

In the ensuing investigation of the crash, the following items were found in the vicinity of the crash. They are listed in order according to the Ohio State Highway Patrol report: left front tire of unit #1 (Rick Fenner's car); left rear tire of unit #1; front tire of unit # 2 (Brandon's 10-speed bike); rear tire of unit #2; eight AA batteries; a six-pack of AA batteries; a pool of blood; a tennis shoe tongue; a wiper blade from unit #1; tennis shoe from unit #2; ball of chewed gum; one cassette tape; one broken cassette tape; debris from the crash (from Fenner's car).

Brandon arrived at University Hospital close to 5 P.M. He was pronounced dead at 23:45 (11:45 P.M.) military time on June 26. He was an organ donor. Later that summer he would have entered the ninth grade at Blanchester High School and played on its football team. "They told us he probably died within 14 minutes after the impact," says Sheree. "He looked awful in the hospital. His head was very swollen. We accepted it when they told us he was brain dead." The Wayne and Goshen Township rescue squads referred Brandon to Air Care. Initial assessment by Air Care was made at 16:53 (4:53 P.M.). An endotracheal tube established an open airway. He was placed on hypovent on 100 percent oxygen. He was noted to be apneic at the scene and completely unresponsive. He was found on his side and became apneic when turned on his back. After intubation, he was taken to University Hospital's emergency department. The death summary by Dr. Barry Cofer stated "The patient had transient hypotension in transit but his blood pressure was noted to be 140 on arrival in fully inflated MAST

Trousers. This decreased to approximately 125 systolic upon deflation. Upon arrival he was tracheally intubated and was without any signs of volitional activity. He had some superficial abrasions to the head and face and had a very large ecchymosis (bruise) and laceration of the left scapular and axillary region." Principal diagnosis was severe closed head injury without return of consciousness. Secondary diagnosis was anoxic brain damage, scapula fracture, and multiple abrasions.

Further, the summary states "The patient was a stocky and muscular white male who was completely unresponsive with cervical collar on and on a backboard. Eyes, ears, nose, and throat (EENT) exam revealed a right forehead abrasion and contusion. The pupils were fixed at 6 mm and equal in diameter. Tympanic membranes were visualized and were clear. Chest had equal bilateral breath sounds. He had a very large abrasion and laceration to the left scapular region and left axillary region without evidence of bleeding. Cardiac exam was regular rhythm without murmur. An abdominal exam revealed he had an old well-healed supraperiumbilical surgical scar caused by a fall on a pop bottle. He had a large left flank contusion. Pelvis was stable to compression. Genitourinary (GU) exam revealed circumcised male with no blood at the meatus. Rectal exam demonstrated poor tone within normal prostrate and was guaiac negative. He had minimal abrasion on the left ankle and otherwise extremities were dry and warm with excellent profusion. Neurologic exam revealed unresponsive to noxious and verbal stimuli. Pupils were equal, round, and fixed at 6 mm. There was no gag reflex and no response to caloric stimulation. Reflexes were flaccid without evidence of deep tendon reflexes or plantar response."

Brandon was taken emergently for a computerized tomography (CT) scan of the head which revealed diffuse edema (serous fluid in connective tissue) with loss of gray white interfacing cisterns as well as left subdural hematoma (hematoma that occurs between the dura mater and arachnoid in the subdural space and that may apply neurologically significant pressure to the cerebral cortex). Open peritoneal lavage in the emergency room was grossly negative and this was confirmed by cell count. He was admitted with the diagnosis of severe closed head injury and left scapular fracture. He preliminarily met the requirements for brain death.

Neurological consultation was obtained and they felt that he indeed met the preliminary requirements for brain death. LifeCenter was notified and arrangements were made for donor status.

A University Hospital social worker, Catherine M. Barney, spoke to Sheree and her family, including Brandon's friends David, Greg, and Paul at 5 P.M. on the 26th. Dr. Jon Getz addressed the family in the emergency room, explaining the six-hour determinants for brain death, legal declaration of death, and broached the subject of donation. Brain death is the total, irreversible cessation of all brain functions including the brain stem. Lack of responsiveness to stimuli, absence of all reflexes, and absence of spontaneous breathing demonstrate it. An electroencephalogram (EEG) or other test may be used by the physician to establish brain death. Brandon was transferred to the surgical intensive care unit (SICU). Sheree's large extended family gathered, including David, who was with Brandon when the accident occurred. Extensive grief and preparatory counseling was provided. The family minister, the Reverend Harmeyer (Baptist), was also with the family. Sheree and her family were anxious with extended delay (after 9 P.M.) to see Brandon. Former transplant coordinator and director of organ procurement Tom Tressler of LifeCenter met with Sheree and the family made the decision to donate Brandon's organs. Tressler was a colleague of mine at LifeCenter for four-and-a half years.

The family remained vigil according to Barney's notes. In the SICU he underwent invasive hemodynamic monitoring. A cardiac echo was obtained which revealed good wall motion without evidence of abnormality except for the possibility of bicuspid aortic valve. However, long discussions with cardiovascular surgery were held and they felt this was not a contraindication to transplant.

Overnight, Brandon developed severe diabetes insipidus as well as disseminated intravascular coagulation. On a respirator, he was maintained with large amounts of hypotonic fluids and blood products and remained relatively stable over night. He was taken to the operating room by the transplant surgery service where he underwent donor cardiectomy, hepatectomy, pancreatectomy, and bilateral nephrectomy. I was called at home at 3 A.M. and arrived at the hospital about 4:30 A.M. Brandon arrived in OR "A" at 10:19 A.M., the procedure began at 10:36 and was finished by 3 P.M. My surgery began at 1 P.M. and ended at 4:30 P.M.

Shortly before the accident June 26, Sheree had been at the grocery store in Blanchester with her friend, Debbie Hughes, David's mother. On their way home, they came upon the accident. "We came out of IGA and I looked at Debbie and said, 'Debbie, let's run by the high school and check on the boys.' I had never done that before. I don't know why I did it. She said, 'Is something wrong?' I said, 'I don't know, I just don't feel right.' We went by the high school and everybody was gone. So we went by the cinema in town and they weren't there either. We went by the sundry store the boys sometimes frequented and their bikes weren't there. We checked everywhere we thought they'd be. Debbie said, 'Is everything OK?' I said, 'I don't know, Debbie, I just don't feel right. I feel like something is wrong.' We were on our way back home and we're going the route the boys usually took, going on 133 and then cutting off on the first road and taking the back roads all the way home. Before we got to that first road they would have taken, we came right up on Brandon lying in the road. We were there before a police officer arrived, before the paramedics. Ours was the second car at the scene."

In Sheree's kitchen that cold, late April Sunday afternoon, I ask Sheree if Brandon would be very happy and proud of the decision she made to donate his organs. "I'm just one of four beneficiaries," I say. "How do you think Brandon feels now?"

"Oh, I think he would feel good about the decision," she says. "He had always said to other people that he was not able to offer much of anything to anybody in his young life. He hadn't made it that far. He gave four people here a chance to go on."

On that April day I was also introduced to Brandon's stepsister and stepbrother, Amanda 10, and Matthew, eight. They had only good memories of their older brother. "I remember he used to lock me out of his room," says a smiling Amanda. She mentions Brandon taught her to play Nintendo. Brandon took her fishing, she remembers. "I caught four fish. I have a picture of that," she recalls proudly. She also tells me she's a cheerleader and she played T-ball. Her mother says she wants to play football next year. "Girls do play," interjects Sheree. There was a girl on Matthew's Pee Wee team.

I ask Matthew if he is sports-oriented. "Football," he says loudly. He has his jersey on, No. 66. He shows me his trophy for the Pee Wee League. "Tell me about your brother," I say. "Tell me the things you did together." Amanda was four and Matthew two when Brandon was killed. "How much do you miss him?" I ask.

He's shy. And that's a tough question. Maybe even a stupid one. Norma intercedes saying he "misses him a lot, just like we all do, don't you honey?"

"Do you think about him a lot?" I ask. He nods shyly. "If he was around, would he give you any advice about playing football?"

"I think he wishes Brandon was here so he could take him out and away from Amanda for awhile," says Sheree with a laugh. Her kids mean everything to her.

"Brandon belonged to all of us," says his grandmother, Norma. "He had a way about him, an air of success. He had a dream of someday playing professional football. He grew a lot from 14 to 15. He was hyperactive but he turned into an adult. He did a complete turnaround. It is hard when you are a kid in a man's body. He was not old enough to handle all his feelings but he opened up and was the most wonderful person. He became an adult. The change was so drastic. Not that there was anything wrong with him to begin with. He turned from a child into a young man."

"He settled down," agrees Sheree.

Sheree and her family are proud of the decision they made to donate Brandon's organs. They still think about Brandon every day. And the pain has not eased. "There are times," says Sheree, "when either of these two (Matthew and Amanda) do little things that remind me of the things Brandon did and I'll call them Brandon. They'll look at me and say, 'Mom, I'm Amanda,' or 'Mom! I'm Matthew, not Brandon.' We do talk about him all the time. It is not a hush, hush subject. As a matter of fact, we have the tape from the *Jerry Springer* show (we were on together with other recipients and transplant professionals in 1991). I work for the nursing home in Blanchester and some of the residents wanted to see it. So I brought it in and we all watched it together and talked about everything. I am very open to discussing it."

Sheree and her family are very close. The day of the accident she arrived at the hospital after 5 P.M. "I had a car full of groceries," she recalls. "Matthew and Amanda were with us," continues Sheree. "I had to get my next door neighbor to watch them. I was in no shape to drive and Debbie was of course worried about David. She was really in no shape to drive either. So my other neighbor offered to take us down. We had to wait for her to get over here. I had to call Ron (Rieke), my stepfather, and my sister. They all lived a lot closer to the hospital so they were already there when I arrived. They had everyone in a little room. Within five minutes after arriving, the doctor came in and told us Brandon was brain dead and that there wasn't anything they could do."

Sheree says the doctor explained everything, and Tom from LifeCenter approached her a little while later to ask about donation. Brandon's heart, liver, and kidneys were donated. On June 27, 1989, in a four-hour operation, I received Brandon's heart. "We were treated well by everyone involved in the donation process," says Sheree.

Hilma Crawford, who in 1989 was the Blanchester Junior High School football coach, and Bob Braman, the varsity head football coach, remember Brandon fondly. Braman has retired from coaching and now teaches science at Blanchester High School. Until recently, Crawford was the varsity head football coach at Clinton Massey High School in Wilmington, Ohio.

"Brandon was a very hard worker," says Crawford. "His goal was to be a football player at Blanchester High School. He was on the offensive line in junior high, but he was pretty skilled and we moved him to running back in the eighth grade. We didn't have a good football team but Brandon worked very hard. I got permission to retire his number (28) and it is in the trophy case at the junior high. At the dedication banquet, his family, including his grandparents, all came. The following year we dedicated the season to him and went 6-1, having one of the best seasons ever at the junior high." When you walk into the main lobby of Blanchester Junior High, one of the first things you see is the trophy case with Brandon's jersey, No. 28.

"I walk by it every day when I go to class," says Braman.

Was Brandon good enough to play varsity in the ninth grade? I ask Crawford and Braman.

"I think he could have," says Crawford. "He was a pretty big kid for junior high. I think he was 6 feet, 185 pounds."

Braman says they were going to try him at defensive end that year.

Brandon had college scholarship potential. His other goals were to join the Air Force or become a police officer. "I think he knew he had scholarship potential and that's why he worked so hard," says Crawford. "He was one of the few kids in the eighth grade that worked hard to become a very good football player. When you ride your bike eight miles one way to the high school to lift weights just for an hour and a half, you're pretty dedicated. We didn't have a whole lot of that dedication."

Braman says that he taught Brandon in junior high science. "He was the same in class as he was for Hilma's football team," reflects Braman. "He worked as hard as he could in the classroom, the same as he did on the football field. He was serious about his studies because he had some serious goals. He did want to play varsity football and I'm sure he wanted to get a college scholarship. He wasn't a straight A student but he did as well as he could with his ability. He was always a neat kid. I was proud of him. I mean, when he completed class every day, and I'm the varsity football coach, and he was a junior high football player, he just had a tendency to come up to me after class and talk about football."

Braman, like Crawford, saw Brandon's ability. Both were waiting for him to develop further.

"He had quite a bit of ability," recalls Braman fondly. "I had talked to him about running track too, that spring. He had not run track the year before. So he was going to do track that spring because I reinforced the idea that it would make him quicker for football. Heaven knows what he could have done in track."

So while Braman had instructed Brandon in the classroom, Crawford taught him four months out of the year for a couple of hours a day.

"The other kids looked up to Brandon," says Crawford with a smile. "I used to use him as an example for my players at Clinton Massey. I think about him. I have some flowers his mom gave me from the funeral. I would bring up his story with the kids I coached.You see kids that are very dedicated in what they are doing, and I bring this story up. Brandon was very dedicated in what he wanted to be. He was also going to get his driver's license. When I'd see a kid today not putting out any effort that reminds me of Brandon because he would always give the maximum effort. To this day, my shoulder still hurts from the day he ran through the shoot at practice we use to keep running backs low. He was just learning to become a running back. I was holding one of the blocking dummies and he missed the dummy and hit me right in the shoulder. At times I can still feel a little pain there and that's from Brandon. He is probably reminding me of it."

Had Brandon been recruited by Moeller, St. Xavier, Colerain, or Cincinnati high schools noted for having top-notch football teams, he probably would have faired pretty well. "He worked his butt off to the point of getting to where he could play so well," says Crawford. "And when you are 6 foot, 185 pounds going into high school, it is hard to tell how much taller he was going to get and how much weight he would have gained. I like to say he was going to be the best player ever. He certainly had the desire."

Brandon was buried at Graceland Memorial Gardens in Milford on June 30, 1989.

The day we visited with Sheree, Amanda, Matthew, and the Riekes, April 23, 1995, was one week after Easter. Six years after my heart transplant, I finally visited Brandon's grave with the Riekes. I thought I would break down and cry as I approached his grave, which was near two blue spruce trees. I did not. The overcast day was bitter cold and rain was in the air. A small brook ran through the cemetery. It felt more like February than April. I looked at Brandon's monument nestled in the ground and gently reached down with Ron's hand trimmer to trim the grass. I lifted the bronze vase delicately from its holder while Debbie placed a half dozen red tulips in it and filled it with water. I admired the decorations. Norma said Matthew had taken on the responsibility of keeping Brandon's grave looking so nice.

I felt a sense of relief. I finally knew Brandon was at peace. And I knew he was smiling down on me every day from heaven. He was my guardian angel. I felt warm inside. I felt close to God. I felt Brandon more that day than ever before.

I had my old Oak Hills High School team jacket on with several of my high school basketball letters. Just for a moment, I was 16 again, driving for the first time, flirting with the girls. It was winter and Brandon and I were shooting baskets in the high school gym. Then we were behind the high school at the football stadium, tossing the football on the freshly mowed grass. It was autumn. Then it was spring and we were warming up on the baseball field. I looked around at the peaceful surroundings as I imagined these things. For seven years during high school and college, I worked summers at a local cemetery. I felt at home here. I felt comfortable. I had been here before. I wanted Brandon to be a part of my life, and in truth he was already a part of my life. Then the blustery wind blew in my face and brought me back to reality. I thought the tears froze on my face. But then I realized there were not any tears, just bottled up emotion looking for a release. I refused to cry. I turned away from Debbie. She had tears in her eyes. I was ashamed I could not cry.

Less than a month later, on May 20, Debbie and I were married. Sheree, Amanda, Matthew, Sheree's sister Brooke, and the Riekes attended the wedding. In a letter postmarked July 21, Sheree made me realize how much a part of my life Brandon is. The letter was addressed to both Debbie and me, but it was in response to Debbie's thank-you note for Sheree's wedding gift.

Dear Debbie & Jeff,

You are more than welcome for the gift certificate. Thank you very much for inviting us to your wedding. It meant more than you know. Thank you for remembering us with the pictures, also. (The wedding photographer took several pictures of us with Sheree and her family.) I know it can be hectic to decorate, but it is also a lot of fun.

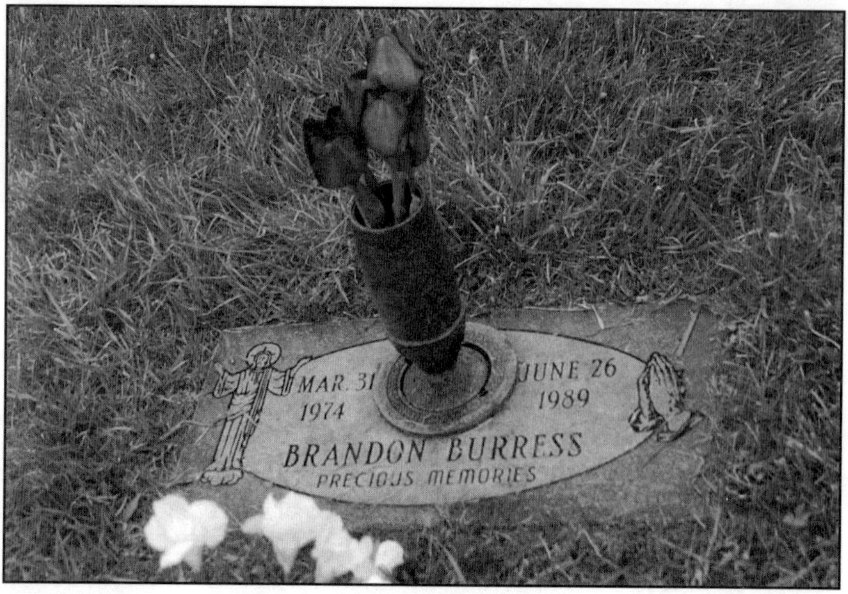

The Ultimate Gift

Brandon's grave at Graceland Memorial Gardens in Milford, Ohio. Debbie and I first visited his grave on April 23, 1995.

Photograph © by Debbie Lueders

Pleased to hear you had a great honeymoon. I'm glad Brandon could give you both so much. Brandon never had a chance to fall in love or get married and I'm glad he was able to give this to someone else. And no one is more deserving.

I (we) couldn't (family also) be more pleased with Jeff receiving Brandon's heart. He is a wonderful person. And you must be also as he chose to spend his life with you. I'm very happy for you both. It makes me feel good to know the two of you are able to enjoy and grow in your life and love together.

The wedding was beautiful. I had very strong and mixed emotions. But everything was great. We did tape the ceremony. This was your day and you chose to include us. It was very hard as I kept feeling this should be Brandon's wedding. Yet, at the same time, I felt Brandon was there and all was okay. I was sad, yet I was happy. I hope you understand what I mean. I want to thank you for remembering Brandon in your wedding program. That was very sweet.

So I hope you and Jeff have a wonderful life together. Enjoy each other and make many, many memories. Please keep in touch and feel free to call anytime. I hope the book goes well as I'm sure it will. If Jeff still wants to talk to David (the boy with Brandon), Jeff may have to pull things out of him but David said he would talk. It seems that everyone forgets David saw it all and how he must feel. This would be very good for him I think. The accident still bothers him a great deal.

Again, best of luck and congratulations in your new life together. I know you both will live it to the fullest. Thank you again.

Warm wishes,

Sheree, Amanda, Matthew

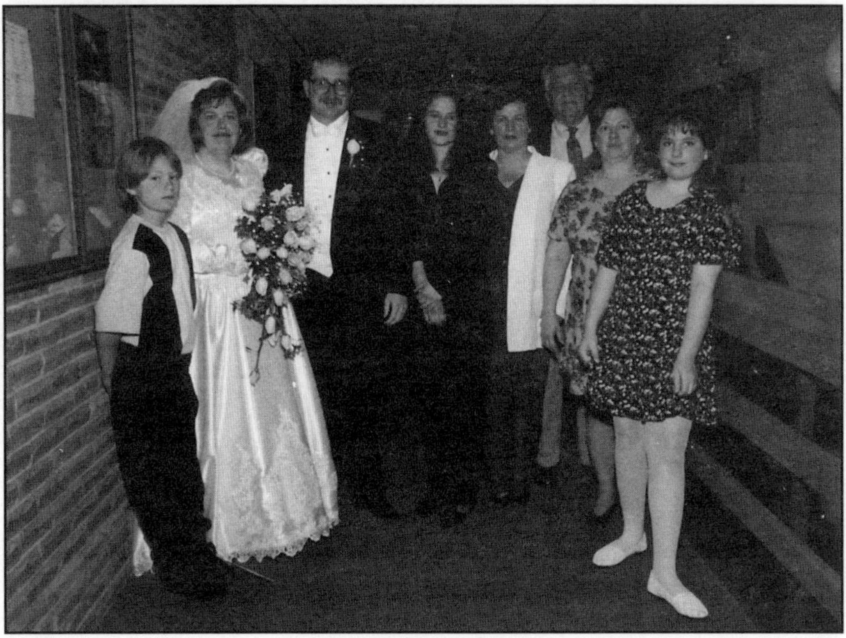

Sharing the "Gift of Life"

My donor family at our wedding on May 20, 1995. *Left to right:* Matthew Gampher, Brandon's stepbrother; Debbie and Jeff Lueders; Brooke Rieke, Sheree Starr's sister; Norma Jean and Ron Rieke, Sheree's mother and stepfather, and Brandon's maternal grandparents; Sheree Starr, Brandon's mother; and Amanda Gampher, Brandon's stepsister.

Photograph © by Lancaster Photography

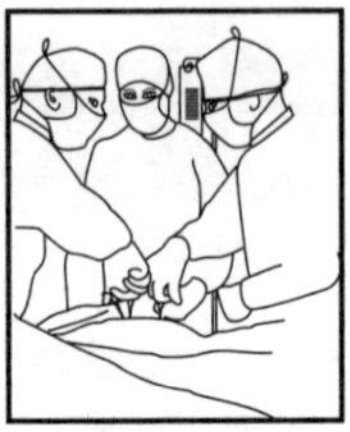

8

Dee Dee Mitten: giving in life, giving in death

It is early evening, July 10, 1995. Debbie and I are following Missy Holliday in our car to the Morrow Cemetery in Morrow, Ohio. On Super Bowl Saturday 1991, Melodee "Dee Dee" Mitten, Missy's younger sister, was killed in a single-car accident minutes from her Morrow home. As we drive into the small but well-kept cemetery, I notice everything: the trees and flowers in bloom, the smell of the grass, the narrow one-lane road that winded around it, enveloping it. It was a very special place. There was solitude. There was sorrow. But there was also a sense of peace.

Dee Dee was Missy's sister, a year younger than her. Missy always referred to her as "my little sister." Missy is a nurse and senior transplant coordinator for LifeCenter. "What do you think when you come out here?" I ask. "What goes through your mind? Do you come out here often?"

"No," she says. "It's just hard for me to come out. I think about Dee Dee all the time, but it's just really hard for me to come here. I come out for Memorial Day and her birthday. Sometimes I like to go if I'm down or thinking about her or having a problem. I go to the cemetery and it makes me feel better. But it's just hard to go."

"Why do you think it's hard?" I ask.

"I just think reality hits and I try not to deal with it and try not to think about it. It just brings back a lot of memories and feelings that I don't care to bring back."

Missy's family is very close. Later that evening at her parents' house in Morrow, they talk about Dee Dee—her life and her death and their decision to donate her organs. Missy's twin sister, Shelly, does not like to talk about Dee Dee's death. Neither she nor her brother, Brian, a musician, was there. Missy's father, Andy, recently retired as loss prevention director at Kings Island, a Midwest amusement park in Kings Mills, Ohio, now owned by Paramount. Now a consultant in loss prevention at Kings Island, Andy is also chief of the Harlan County Fire and Rescue Department. Her mother, Diane, works for a graphic design firm in Cincinnati.

Diane and Andy begin to talk with pride about Dee Dee. I knew very little about her except what Missy had told me at the office.

"I could start by telling you that my mother always said Dee Dee came out with a smile on her face," says Diane, wiping the tears away. "She was always smiling. She was the most outgoing of our four kids. She was always so friendly from the time she was a little girl. She always made it a point to speak to people first. She wasn't the least bit inhibited by adults, and from the time she was real small she was very active in school." Diane goes on to say that at Morrow Elementary School, from the time Dee Dee was in the second or third grade, she was active in school plays and musicals.

In high school at Little Miami, she was in cheerleading for four years and was homecoming queen in 1984. She played soccer and softball in high school and was vice president of her senior class. "She was always involved in activities and had so many friends," says Andy. She was so outgoing but not necessarily outspoken.

After high school, she attended Addison Community College in Fort Myers, Florida, and received an associate degree in criminal justice. Then she continued her education at the University of South Florida in Tampa. Then she decided to change her career and came home to attend Raymond Walters (a college of the University of Cincinnati) to study dental hygiene.

Andy and Diane still question why this accident happened to Dee Dee. Andy says he can't say Dee Dee was the best of the kids, but she was the most outgoing and friendly, the one who was going to be somebody. "She wanted to be someone different," says Andy. "At her fifth-year high school class reunion she was active in organizing and putting the program out," Andy recalls.

It was a Saturday afternoon in January. The day before the 1991 Super Bowl. Dee Dee was working as a waitress at DeSha's, a Montgomery restaurant very close to her home. She had been working there since it opened and she was always real crazy about the place and people who worked there. Andy says she made a lot of friends there. Dee Dee had been home that day studying for exams on Monday. She had to be at work at 4 P.M. It had been very cold and snowy. A lot of ice patches remained on the roads. Her boyfriend, Brian Gabbard, had been at the house. He came out since he wasn't going to be able to go out with her that evening. He spent a couple of hours with her. "He told us after the fact that when Dee Dee hugged him good-bye he thought to himself the hug was more special than any other ones that she had given him," recalls Diane. He left the house right behind her.

Dee Dee's car was a white Ford EXP that Diane and Andy had bought for her when she was in school in Florida. "It was her car and it had Florida plates on it until right before we finally changed it over because we knew she wasn't going back to Florida until after she finished Raymond Walters," says Andy. "I think she still had hopes to go back down there after dental hygiene school. She loved Florida. She had so many friends that she had made over the years down there."

Dee Dee left the house with her dog, Max, an Alaskan husky who liked to chase cars, following behind her. He was her dog. She backed out of the driveway and when Max went after her car she threw him some dog biscuits and then drove up the road. "Brian was driving my truck," says Andy. There was another car behind Dee Dee and then Brian. She was about 1/2 mile from the house. There were some curves in the road. There was snow and ice. There had been some melting and the water had drained down these driveways across the road which made it icy. She was at a curve and was running a little late for work. "Not real late," remembers Andy, "but close to being late."

"I'm sure she was probably speeding," says Missy, "but knowing her she was probably leaning down to put make-up on or doing something else and lost control of the car. She had fastened her seat belt and was a very careful driver."

Dee Dee went around the curve and lost it. She hit a patch of ice and her car slid sideways into a tree. She hit on the driver's side. Andy says she was the best of all the kids about wearing her seat belt. "A head-on impact she might have survived," says Andy, "but this was sideways into a tree that was huge. It was the only tree on the road that big. Brian came upon the accident. We were living on Edwardson Road then. I remember I was sitting in the chair on Super Bowl weekend watching some kind of football show. Brian had my truck and I remember hearing the siren and seeing the red light turned on. He was blowing the siren as he came down the road. I remember hearing the siren but it didn't sink in until he came in the house." It was only minutes later when he came running in the front door screaming, "Dee's been in an accident."

Missy was at her parents' house. Both she and her dad knew the accident was serious by Brian's tone. Missy ran to the telephone to dial 911 but Andy said he would call on his radio. He called the Harlan County Fire Department to dispatch its life squad. "The county later told us they had gotten a 911 hang-up," recalls Andy.

Diane had just lost her father and was visiting her sister. On the way home, she came upon the accident. Brian, Missy, and Andy were the only ones there. "When I first saw the cars, there was a big light there and I didn't see Dee Dee's car," says Diane. "The first thing that ran through my mind was that somebody had slid off the road and gone into the lake. When I got around the curve, I saw her car. I just stopped my car in the middle of the road and took off running toward her car. A neighbor came out and grabbed me. She said, 'They're taking care of her. Why don't we go back to the house.' So she took me back to the house. I got on the telephone and called the rest of the kids. I didn't know anything at that point, but I knew in my heart it was bad because I saw where the car was and the tree that Dee Dee hit."

Andy was chief of the Harlan County Fire Department and Missy was on the squad. "We got to the scene and saw the car against the tree," remembers Andy. "Then, we saw Dee Dee. She was still breathing and had no visible injuries. She was unconscious. Missy got into the car and as soon as I got in I checked her. Her pulse was rapid."

"Although her pulse was real thready, she had a good blood pressure at the scene," recalls Missy. During the several minutes before Air Care arrived, I talked to Dee Dee and told her everything was going to be all right. I felt helpless. There was nothing else I could do but pray."

Dee Dee was trapped in the car, so after Andy called for Air Care the rest of the rescue equipment arrived on the scene. "I cannot remember what conversation took place then," says Andy. "I just remember trying to figure out how we were going to get her out of the car and what to do next. Missy stayed in the car the whole time. We tried to keep her warm. I don't remember the temperature but it was very cold. It had to be well below freezing, maybe close to zero. It was about 4:30 P.M."

Dee Dee had worn a real heavy coat, but she wasn't moved until the Hurst tools arrived. She had to be cut out. The back seat was pulled down and eventually she was pulled out the back. The squad had arrived by then, and she had a C-collar put on and was placed on a backboard and taken out the back of the car. After Air Care arrived, Dee Dee was put in the squad and driven five hundred feet to Air Care's landing site. The paramedic and doctor on board Air Care got into the squad.

"I talked to them there," says Andy. "They went to work on her. She had no visible injuries. She had multiple injuries but they were not visible at the time. You could tell by looking at her that things were not going real well. But I still didn't believe it was that serious."

Dee Dee was flown to University Hospital in Cincinnati. By the time the family made the 45-minute trip to the hospital from the accident scene, an emergency room (ER) physician came out and said, "It doesn't look good." These were the words of Dr. Daniel Storer, director of emergency medical service at the hospital. "I had met him before," says Andy, "but I didn't know him very well."

"We were devastated," recalls Missy. I asked God, "How can you do this to us? Our family had already suffered more than our fair share of tragedy. I couldn't fathom the thought of now having to give up my sister. In my mind, I was not going to let it happen. I handled the situation worse than anyone in my family. I ran out the ER doors screaming. I wanted to run away. It doesn't make sense, but I just wanted to run away. I didn't care if I ever knew, if I ever saw her again, I didn't want to know if she died. I didn't want to deal with never seeing her again. I didn't want to face the truth. I felt helpless. But I had to face the fact that Dee Dee might not make it."

The other tragedy that Missy mentions was the death in November 1987 of her grandmother from injuries she suffered in a house fire. Myrtle Kemp was 87 years old and very healthy. A kerosene heater caught fire and her grandfather, Henry, dragged it through the kitchen door. "My mom was actually pulling in their driveway when the fire began," says Missy. "Then the house exploded. My mom and grandfather ran around the house trying to find my grandmother. They could not. She died of smoke inhalation. My grandfather felt so guilty. He lived with us for a year and a half until my parents built the house they are living in now for him. He died three years later from a massive heart attack."

Four days after my grandma died, one of my parents' best friends was killed in an airplane crash half a mile from our house. "My dad and I were on that scene too," says Missy. "It was my mom's best friend's husband."

Dee Dee was transferred from the ER to the surgical intensive care unit (SICU) at University Hospital. "We waited, praying for a miracle," says Missy. "I can remember making many deals with God that night. However, at midnight, my dad gathered us together and told us that the doctors had performed a brain death test and it showed Dee Dee had no brain function." They said she would not live through the night. Her brain was going to swell. It was about 5:30 A.M.

"Shortly after this, a resident walked out of Dee Dee's room to speak with us," remembers Missy. "He brought up the possibility of organ and tissue donation. He was somewhat cold and insensitive. He did not seem sympathetic to the fact that we had just been told this devastating news. But we felt very close to Dee Dee's nurses. Through them, we decided to consider this option. We all knew that Dee Dee, if ever given the chance, would want to help others in this way." Dee Dee lived about 15 hours after the accident.

At 7 A.M., after the second brain death exam, Ron Dreffer, a transplant coordinator and former executive director of LifeCenter, came to the hospital and talked to the family about donation. "He answered our questions and explained what would happen at this point," says Missy. "We signed the consent form, said our good-byes to Dee Dee, and left the hospital.

"We knew donation was something Dee Dee would have wanted," says Diane. "There was no doubt. The only thing I said I didn't want to donate was her eyes. I couldn't bring myself to do that." Dee Dee died on January 27, 1991. The cause of death was blunt trauma to the head (closed head injury).

The night of Dee Dee's visitation it was raining and cold. More than one thousand people attended the visitation. "We live in a small town," says Diane. "It was the biggest funeral they ever had. Some of the older

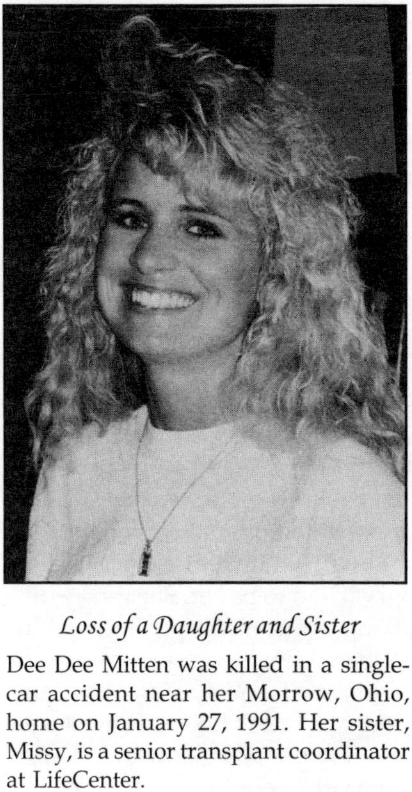

Loss of a Daughter and Sister

Dee Dee Mitten was killed in a single-car accident near her Morrow, Ohio, home on January 27, 1991. Her sister, Missy, is a senior transplant coordinator at LifeCenter.

Photograph © by Diane Mitten

people—relatives and friends—could not stand outside in that heavy rain. So many people loved Dee Dee. She touched many lives."

Months after Dee Dee's death, Diane received a letter from a woman she did not know. "I wouldn't know who she was today, but Dee Dee had waited on her and her husband at DeSha's. She went in the restaurant and asked to sit in Dee Dee's section. The restaurant manager told them Dee Dee had died. She wrote me the neatest letter. It said what a sweet girl she was and how she and her husband had grown to love her in a short period of time. She was always so friendly. That letter meant so much to me because to this day, I don't know who these people are. But they took the time to write me and tell me what they thought of her. Dee Dee was special and not because she was ours. She was just a special child."

Dee Dee's heart went to a young Cincinnati woman. One of the kidney recipients also was from Cincinnati. A young girl from Dayton, Ohio, received her other kidney. The liver recipient was from Columbus, Ohio.

For Missy, time passed very slowly after Dee Dee's death. She returned to Indianapolis to work as a nurse. Within six months, she returned to Cincinnati working at Children's Hospital Medical Center (CHMC) in the cardiac intensive care unit (CICU). In September 1993, she accepted a position as a transplant coordinator at LifeCenter. She left after two years but returned to LifeCenter in 1997.

"I now look at my sister's life as a gift that was given to those of us who knew and loved her. Although her time on this earth was brief, I learned more from her in that short period of time than I could learn from anyone in a lifetime. I feel honored that I can say, 'She was my sister.'"

Dee Dee always did the unexpected. "She was a practical joker," recalls Andy. "When she was living in Florida, she worked for People's Express. She could fly wherever she wanted to go. Generally, she would show up on our front porch. She was full of surprises. She'd come home on the weekend and work something out with her sisters. Our sister-in-law lived across the street. She'd tell them to pick her up at the airport so she could surprise her mother. We wouldn't see her for two or three months, and then all of a sudden she'd just show up and say, 'Here I am.'"

Missy says that Dee Dee was just a great person. "I know a lot of people say this about people they lose," she says. "But everybody loved her. She never judged anybody. She always looked at the better side of a person. She was always optimistic. I have a ton of memories—ice-skating on my parents' lake, Christmases. The last night we had together, the night before she died, was probably my favorite memory. We hooked up with a mutual friend from Indianapolis, Dee Dee's best friend. We went out. I had not seen her friend in about a year. We had the best time. Dee Dee asked me to sing in her wedding that night. I kind of feel she knew something was going to happen. I don't know if she really did."

After Dee Dee died, Missy questioned God and was bitter. "I was very mad. Part of me put the accident out of my mind. I got really angry right after it happened. I was never angry with her but I was very angry about the fact she had to be the one to die when there are people in this world that really make nothing of themselves. Not that that makes it right for them to die either, but I was very angry it had to be her. She was getting her life together and was so happy, talking about marriage. It just didn't seem fair. Then I went through a stage where I finally accepted her death. I was thankful that she wasn't murdered or raped. I really didn't have anybody to blame. I was so thankful a drunk driver didn't hit her. When I went to her car, I know she was unconscious, but I'm pretty sure she didn't know what hit her. That gives me a sense of comfort."

The Mittens have a scholarship in her name at Raymond Walters College, a branch of the University of Cincinnati. It is a yearly scholarship that goes to freshmen. There is also a softball tournament held each May in her honor. It is called the Dee Dee Mitten Memorial Softball Tournament. The funds raised are used to purchase equipment for the athletic association.

A monument at the park symbolizes Dee Dee's love for life and the people in it:

In memory of Dee Dee Mitten
whose passion for life filled
all of her 23 years.
Her Love will be forever felt by
those of us whom she touched.

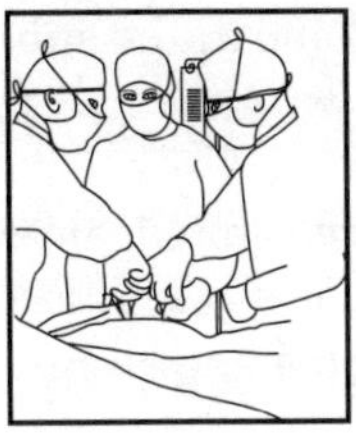

9

Randy Ruwan: a gifted athlete, a caring person

An excerpt from "The Final Act" (*Cincinnati Enquirer*, December 26, 1995) by John Johnston:

> The photo was enlarged from a small snapshot and now hangs on a wall in the den. It's Bev Ruwan's favorite picture of her son, Randy.
>
> *It shows a handsome young man in a red V-neck sweater striking a happy, relaxed, confident pose. Hands are clasped behind a head of short, blond hair, and there's that big smile.*
>
> *How typical. Randy almost always wore a smile.*
>
> *When the picture was snapped on Thanksgiving Day, 1992, he seemingly had much to be thankful for. A star athlete while at Elder High School, he was in the second year of a baseball scholarship at an Illinois college, with hopes of being drafted by a pro team. He made his best grades that fall.*
>
> *A month later, on Dec. 23, Randy returned to his parents' Bridgetown home for the holidays. Sitting in the living room on Christmas Eve with his mother, father and younger sister, flashing that familiar smile, he declared, 'This is the best Christmas ever.'*
>
> *A few hours later, he walked into the garage. He got behind the steering wheel of his pale gray Mustang. He started the engine. And then, instead of driving to an aunt's house to join the rest of his family, he sat there. Inhaling carbon monoxide.*

In 1992, Randy Ruwan seemed to have it all. He was a student and baseball player in his second year at Triton College, a junior college in River Grove, Illinois, not far from Chicago. Triton had the reputation for attracting pro baseball scouts. He was in the second year of a baseball scholarship. A southpaw, he played right field and batted left-handed. Several pro baseball scouts were interested in him. At 5 feet, 9 inches and 180 pounds with short blond hair, Randy was good looking, well liked by his friends, both male and female, and he seemed to love everyone. He had graduated from Elder High School in Cincinnati, playing on both the football and baseball teams.

But on Christmas Eve 1992, Randy sat in his pale gray 5-liter 1988 Mustang in the two-car garage of his parents' Cincinnati home in the suburb of Bridgetown. The car's engine was running and the windows were down. The garage doors were closed. He died two days later at University Hospital in Cincinnati. He was 19. He left a short, handwritten suicide note on the passenger seat: *Mom and Dad. I love you. I'll always love you. It was nothing you said or did, but a struggle within myself.* His organs and tissues were donated.

He had come home for Christmas vacation from Triton on Wednesday, December 23. His father, Ralph, in his late 40s, is a short, but well-built man. He has been a Cincinnati police officer for more than 20 years. His mother, Bev, is 48. She sells real estate for Coldwell Banker/West Shell. She is a loving, caring person, who hugs me every time I see her. Her tears come easily when she talks about Randy. But then she seems to smile through those tears as she and Ralph still ask themselves why it happened and why they didn't see it coming. They have been married for more than 30 years. I spoke to them both on an October evening in 1995 in the den of the spacious, well-decorated home they built in 1989 in Bridgetown. Their daughter, Tracy, was expecting her first child then. Their granddaughter, Kayla, was born November 10, 1995. Kayla is now four and has an eight-month-old brother, Nicholas Randall. Bev says he looks exactly like Randy.

The day after Randy got home was Christmas Eve, a Thursday. "We had our Christmas around 4 P.M. on Christmas Eve," recalls Bev vividly. "And then we went to my sister's house. We had to be there by 6:30 P.M. Randy went his way and we all went our separate ways. He was going to meet us later at my sister's. That was not to happen."

"Randy wanted to take a whirlpool bath," interjects Ralph. "We had some free weights and workout equipment downstairs near his bedroom. The whirlpool was down there too."

"Everybody had their showers and we were all getting ready to go," says Bev. "He gave Tracy a kiss good-bye because she left early to take my sister's kids to see Santa Claus. We knew we were going to meet up with him later at my sister's. Nothing was really out of the ordinary until he didn't show up. It was getting later and later. We thought he was at his girlfriend's and his girlfriend thought he was with us. So really, he was pretty slick."

His girlfriend wasn't with the Ruwans at Bev's sister's. She was supposed to be. They were going to be coming together. "That is where the mix-up was and we didn't really know it. My sister talked to Randy at 7 P.M. and I talked to him at 7:30 P.M. His girlfriend talked to him at 7:45 P.M.

She was the last one to talk to him. We figured this (suicide) roughly happened at 8:50 or 9 P.M. By the time Ralph got back to the house it was 9 P.M."

Ralph returned to the house. "I thought he had fallen asleep in the whirlpool," says Ralph.

"We really thought he had drowned," concurs Bev.

When Ralph returned home, he could hear Randy's car running in the garage. He ran in the house and hit the garage door opener and saw Randy sitting in his car. "I tried to wake him up," says Ralph, holding back tears. "But there was no response. He was unconscious. I dragged him out of the car and took him outside on the driveway." According to Johnston's article, Randy was wearing a new turtleneck and sweater he had gotten as Christmas gifts a few hours earlier. At first, Ralph thought Randy might have passed out. "He was kind of gasping but still was breathing." Ralph called 911 and the Green Township/Mack Fire Department responded within minutes, as it was right up the road from the Ruwans' house.

"We kept calling from my sister's but the line was busy," explains Bev. "Finally I got through and Ralph said he had called the life squad. He told us that Randy tried to kill himself. We went to Mercy Franciscan Hospital-Western Hills Campus and from there Randy was Air Cared to University Hospital in Cincinnati, a trauma hospital. His heart stopped at Mercy Franciscan Hospital-Western Hills Campus. They brought him back and then they Air Cared him right away to University."

At University Hospital, the Ruwans were told Randy was brain dead. Bev says she had to initiate the discussion of organ and tissue donation with the neurosurgeon who told her that Randy was brain dead. She and Ralph were then approached by a transplant coordinator from LifeCenter to discuss organ and tissue donation. "It was not a hard decision to make," says Ralph.

"We knew this was the only way he could live on," explains Bev. "I had been thinking, Well, if we're going to lose him, I'd like to see others live. That brought me comfort. We had met with the transplant coordinator several times at the hospital and knew Randy was brain dead and it was a matter of time before the man upstairs was going to take him. We decided donation was the best thing to do. It's what Randy would have wanted. And what better gift than the 'gift of life' could Randy have given, especially at Christmas."

"I look differently at organ and tissue donation than I did before," Tracy says. "When it is your brother laying there, you want to be able to help someone else. Since Randy's death, I feel good that someone else is living with his organs and tissues. I feel a part of him is still here, that he's not completely gone. I'm glad others have the chance to live. I'm happy for them."

Ralph and Bev knew the type of kid Randy had been. "He was always helping people," recalls Ralph fondly. "In high school, there was one kid that nobody wanted to have anything to do with. He was kind of an outcast. Randy started hanging out with him and all of a sudden everybody started liking this kid." Teachers at Elder would take him with them on retreats to talk to underclassmen about peer pressure and other topics. "We knew being a donor is something he would have wanted," says Ralph.

"So why did Randy do it?" I ask. "What precipitated this? He must have known this would be traumatic to the entire family, especially at Christmas time."

"We don't know," says Ralph stoically.

"We are still trying to figure out why he committed suicide," says Bev tearfully. "Trust me, there is not a day goes by that I don't sit around and ask why. Some days I think I have an answer. But I never do."

"Something on Triton's team?" I ask.

"He had been red-shirted his freshman year and this was only the beginning of his sophomore year," says Bev. "I don't know. Several pro baseball scouts had scouted him the year before. He was an awesome athlete. Whatever this was..."

Ralph says they really don't know what happened at Triton his sophomore year. "It wasn't even baseball season yet. Bev believes it may have had something to do with the team." He had a girlfriend at Triton and one near his home, though his mother insists he was not a player.

"He was the type of kid who would not go to proms because he wouldn't want to pick between girls," says Bev. He didn't want to hurt the girls' feelings so he would not go. He was very popular. Ralph and Bev continue to believe a woman was not to blame for his suicide.

Randy's paternal grandfather, Tom Ruwan, died of cancer in 1992. According to Johnston's *Enquirer* article he had a 15-month battle with cancer. The Ruwans found out after Randy's death that Randy was spending a lot of time at the cemetery where his grandfather was buried. "We did not know this," concedes Bev. "I think a lot of things just got to Randy. I don't think it was any one thing. Maybe it was baseball and a combination of other things."

A year before Randy's death he had an episode of rectal bleeding. He had gone to the doctor right before Christmas and he thought he had cancer then. "He was a health fanatic," maintains Bev. He received a call from the doctor saying it was just a muscle strain from lifting weights. He was told to lay off the weights and the bleeding would stop. The next year, he was still bleeding. Johnston's article says: "On December 22—two days before that fateful Christmas Eve—Randy called home from Triton College. He was crying. He told his mother he knew he was dying."

I said, "What are you talking about?" recalls Bev. "You know what the doctor told you. And then he told me it had stopped. If it had just stopped the week he called me, that was not going to help him. I really believe he thought something was seriously wrong with him. So he was getting out of here before we had to watch him die like we did Grandpa Ruwan. Maybe he wanted to spare us. Ralph's mom believes that too. We are still trying to figure out why."

Ralph and Bev try to cope every day with Randy's death. "Every day you think about it," says Ralph. "There is not one day that you don't think about it and I guess there never will be."

"You have to carry on," maintains Bev.

On their decision to donate Randy's organs and tissues, Ralph says he "can understand a lot of times the recipients feel bad or guilty because their life is at the cost of another. It's really not at the cost of another; the other person was already gone. They are just fortunate enough to get their life back. We don't want the recipients to feel bad. We want them to feel good so we can feel good. The whole idea is that if they as recipients are not happy, then there really wasn't much sense in donating to them. It should be a happy moment for them, not a sad one. The sad moment was when we lost our son. The happy moment is that someone doesn't have to lose a son or daughter like we did. I have never been in a position where I faced end-stage organ failure and needed a transplant or I would die. My former partner's wife, Sharon Ruberg, is a kidney/pancreas recipient. She had diabetes. She is making it, and they have two children."

Several recipients who received Randy's organs have responded in writing to the Ruwans. LifeCenter maintains donor and recipient confidentiality. Recipients or donor families may, however, write to LifeCenter. The letters are then forwarded to the donor family or recipient with no names being exchanged. If they wish to continue to correspond mutually and even meet, they may do so. LifeCenter is usually involved in the first meeting.

Cincinnatian Bill Tarter received Randy's heart. The Ruwans met him in 1994 on Randy's 21st birthday. His wife died of cancer several months after the meeting. He has two children.

The Ruwans were the first Cincinnati donor family to attend the National Donor Recognition Ceremony in Washington, D.C., April 17, 1994. That year, the first it was held, was in memory of Nancy Moore Thurmond, late daughter of Senator Strom Thurmond (D-South Carolina). "We definitely think families need to discuss organ and tissue donation ahead of time, before they're in a crisis like we were," said the Ruwans in 1994.

Bev joined Self-Support for Bereaved Parents shortly after Randy's death. The group is for parents whose children have died – most from suicide. It meets at Shiloh United Methodist in Delhi.

Bev has found the support group to be very helpful. Ralph has not. "He went a couple of times and said it wasn't for him," says Bev. "But it helps me. We have Christmas parties and memorials."

Twice a year Bev talks to Tom Darnell's religion classes at Elder for a week on depression and also to Seton High School (a girls' Catholic high school) religion classes. "My manager at the office knows I am really committed to this," says Bev. "His son played baseball with Randy. This is two weeks out of my year that I really feel good about. One of the times is right before Christmas. The other is in April. The kids sometimes write letters. We figure if we only help one kid then we've done our job."

Randy is buried in Old St. Joseph Cemetery in Price Hill on West Eighth Street. Ralph used to patrol there and he'd visit Randy's grave every day. "He wouldn't admit it at first," says Bev. Ralph now works for internal affairs with the Cincinnati police.

"Is it a comfort?" I ask.

"Yeah, sometimes," says Ralph.

"Do you ever feel angry at Randy for doing this?" I ask them both. "You must still question why he did it with so much going for him?"

"You don't know how many times we've asked why," replies Ralph.

"I have never been angry at Randy for taking his own life," says Bev tearfully. "The only anger I have with him was what he said to Tracy (Randy joked about how people try to kill themselves and can't even do it right.) According to Johnston's article, Bev learned from his Triton roommates that Randy had discussed carbon monoxide poisoning that fall, but not in the context of killing himself. "It's not really anger," maintains Bev. "I guess because I'm his mom and I have never felt anger towards him. The way I look at it, he was sick. We really missed the depression. That was the hardest thing to deal with. As parents, we missed the depression and all signs in between. This didn't just happen overnight."

Randy did not seem to show any outward signs of depression. "That's why he did it the day after he came home," surmises Bev. "I had a doctor's appointment for him the next week to see our family physician. I knew if there was something physically wrong with him the doctor would detect it." Bev says she knew something was not right with Randy even though she did not see any signs or evidence of a depression.

Bev proudly points to the fact that besides being an awesome athlete he was a neat, caring, loving person.

Ralph says he was meticulous about everything. His father would pitch to him for hours on the fields of Western Hills High School until he got his swing down just right, hitting the ball on the "sweet" spot of the bat each time, with tape on the bat marking that "sweet" spot. According to Ralph, Randy's "clothes had to be perfect. His shoes had to be perfect. His hair had to be perfect. He kept his hair short but he'd comb his hair longer than you or me. His car. We'd clean his car and I'm real particular keeping my car clean. Well, I'd help him clean his car and he'd spend another hour or two to make sure the engine was clean. He'd clean the windows. When you clean the windows with newspaper and Windex it keeps all the streaks off. He'd clean it and clean it until there were no streaks. Everything had to be perfect. And I always thought that was good. Now I'm starting to think he wanted everything too perfect. Maybe it finally caught up with him. If something didn't go the way he wanted it, deep down it probably bothered him."

In the basement bar of the Ruwans' Bridgetown home is one of Randy's baseball jerseys. Framed, it dominates the paneled wall. It is a Chambers Hautman team jersey, Randy's old American Legion team. On one sleeve is the American Legion emblem. On the other is the American flag. At the bottom right-hand corner are Randy's batting gloves.

Dick Kuehn, a veteran baseball coach on Cincinnati's west side, began the Randy Ruwan Memorial Tournament over the Fourth of July weekend in 1995. The four-day tournament involves six American Legion teams, three local and three from out of town. It is a five-game round robin with the four top teams playing on Sunday for the championship.

Kuehn says he went to Ralph and Bev Ruwan to seek permission to have the tournament. They were all for it.

Kuehn met Randy through his (Kuehn's) son, Brad, who had coached Randy in a baseball program at Western Hills High School, and through Chambers Hautman. "He and Brad got along well," recalls Kuehn. "Randy loved Brad's coaching. They got along well because they were both intense competitors."

Mark Thompson is the current varsity baseball coach at Elder High School. He came to Elder in 1990, Randy's junior year. "When I first started coaching, my son was about three years old," remembers Thompson. "Randy was his hero. He really got along well with small kids. We used to do parish clinics and camps, working with their kids for a day. Randy loved helping out at these. He always did really well in anything having to do with kids. And these kids seemed to be drawn to him."

Thompson says Randy was extremely meticulous. "He was a lot like his father in that respect," notes Thompson. "He (Randy) was always the best-dressed kid on road trips. His uniform, too, always had to be just right."

When I ask Thompson if he thinks Randy could have gone pro in baseball, he only says, "I don't know." Thompson is very candid. "He was a year removed from me. You never know how a kid is going to develop. He had the ability, but he was his own worst enemy. The biggest thing about Randy was that he had trouble leaving his last at bat. So if he would strike out or pop up, he was frustrated. He was a perfectionist. He wanted to hit the ball hard every time. And he did most of the time. If he made an out but hit the ball hard, that was fine. He was a pretty good player. If he could have prepared himself mentally for every time at bat, I think he had a chance to turn pro. Now we will never know. He had a good arm, he was pretty quick, he had good power, and he hit the ball to all fields. He had a good shot of signing a professional contract."

When Randy attempted suicide, the Ruwans called Thompson to come to University Hospital. Randy was on a respirator. "I was there for a couple of hours with his family," recalls Thompson sadly. "Everyone was in shock."

"I think everybody at Elder came to the funeral home," says Thompson. "Everybody who knew must have come. He was that kind of kid. He was very charismatic. He had a lot of friends. The line for the viewing was just unbelievable. "I didn't have an answer as to why Randy would do this," says Thompson candidly. A lot of people had trouble grasping why he would do it. Who knows?"

One of Randy's final requests was to be buried in his Elder baseball uniform. Thompson complied. "It was a rough situation," remembers Thompson. "I knew how much baseball meant to him."

Thompson says Randy was always "a super determined kid. He was determined in everything he did. If he set his sight on a goal, he was going to go through walls to try and attain that goal."

Thompson also recalls Randy being a very solid student. "He wasn't one who struggled in the classroom," says Thompson.

Though Thompson has blocked out many memories of Randy, perhaps because they were as close as a player and coach can get, he does recall one baseball story when he coached Randy at Chambers Hautman.

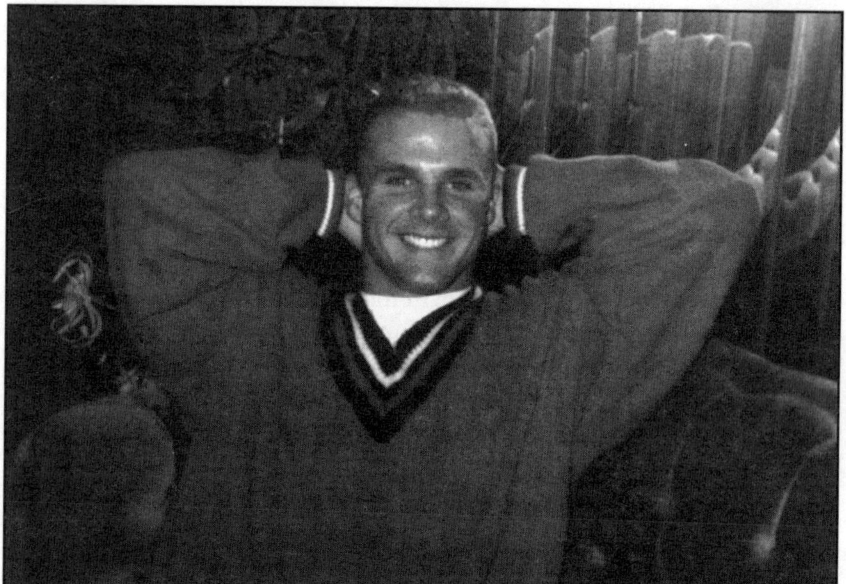

Remembering a Son

In one of the last photographs taken of him, Randy Ruwan's smile and relaxed pose are caught on camera. The photograph was taken on Thanksgiving Day 1992, at the Ruwan's house in Bridgetown, a Cincinnati suburb.

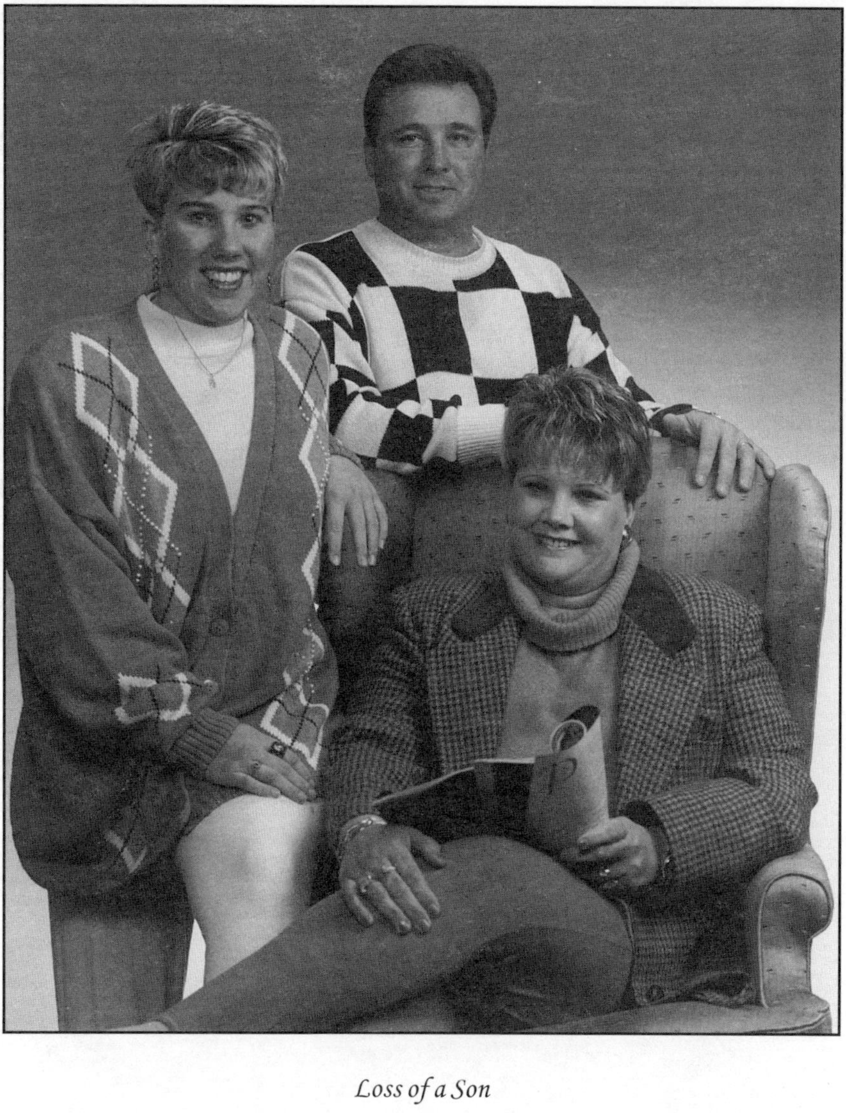

Loss of a Son

A photograph of Tracy, Ralph, and Beverley Ruwan of Cincinnati used in educational brochures and other material for LifeCenter, the organ procurement organization for Greater Cincinnati. Randy Ruwan, their son and Tracy's brother, was an outstanding athlete at Triton College in Illinois. He died December 26, 1992, and was an organ and tissue donor. The Ruwans attended the first National Donor Recognition Ceremony in Washington, D.C., in April 1993. They are LifeCenter volunteers.

Photograph © by Binstadt Photography

"My one regret is that we (Chambers Hautman) were in the semifinals of the American Legion Tournament that summer (1991), Randy's senior year. I had Randy coming up to the plate and I sent the runners. It was a first and third situation and we tried a double steal. The kid on third got thrown out at the plate to end the game. Randy had been on a hot hitting streak throughout the tournament; he played terrific baseball. Thinking back, it was a stupid play on my part. I had a hot hitter up and a very determined kid. He would have found a way to get the job done. Maybe I overcoached. Randy's season and high school career were done at that point. Goddamned, I should have let the kid hit. He was swinging a hot bat."

Ralph, Bev, and Tracy Ruwan remain fervent supporters of organ and tissue donation. They were featured in a poster for Greater Cincinnati hospital healthcare professionals and in church and synagogue bulletin inserts for *National Donor Sabbath,* which promotes organ and tissue donation in November. Their photo is currently being used in the public and professional displays of LifeCenter. They continue to volunteer their time and services at LifeCenter.

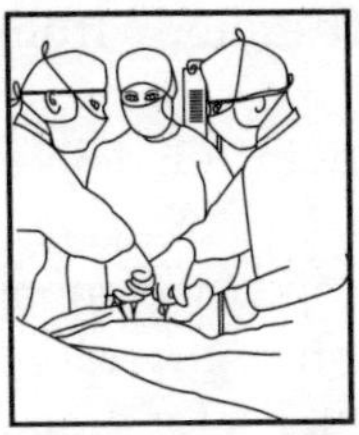

10

Peg Werling: life was important to her

West Chester, Ohio, residents Joseph Werling and his family, stepdaughters Carrie, Stephanie, and Tracy Whittum, and daughters Nicole and Michelle, were among two hundred donor family members from around the country who visited Washington, D.C., April 2, 1995, to commemorate loved ones who were organ and tissue donors. It was the second annual National Donor Recognition Ceremony, co-sponsored by the Division of Organ Transplantation (DOT), local organ and tissue procurement agencies and national transplant-related organizations. The Werlings represented all organ and tissue donor families for 1994 in Greater Cincinnati. Their trip was sponsored by LifeCenter, Ohio Valley Tissue and Skin Center, and the Cincinnati Eye Bank for Sight Restoration Inc.

Since 1985, one week each year has been designated by the president as a time to pay tribute to these individuals and families, and to call public attention to the critical need for donors. National Organ and Tissue Donor Awareness Week (NOTDAW) was April 16–22. In 1995 the ceremony occurred several weeks before NOTDAW. Among the other donor families who attended this ceremony were both the donor and recipient parents (Martin and Julee Erkela, and Sherrie and Lonnie Maize, respectively) featured in a 1995 television documentary, "A Heart for Olivia." Chester Szuber, 58, of Berkley, Michigan, who received his daughter Patti's heart when she was killed in an automobile accident near Knoxville, Tennessee, also attended. Szuber's transplant was performed at William Beaumont Hospital in Royal Oak, Michigan, on August 22. She was 22. Californians Reginald and Maggie Green, and daughter, Eleanor, also attended. The Greens donated son Nicholas' organs and tissues after bandits killed him in a holdup attempt in Italy in 1994 where he and his family were traveling.

Press coverage in Italy and throughout the world was intense after the Greens donated Nicholas' organs and tissues. Reports of the Greens' gift galvanized the Italian population that, at the time, had the lowest donor rate of any industrialized nation. Since the donation, Italians have responded with their own outpouring of generosity, and donation rates have already increased by 20 percent as a direct result of what is now being called the "Nicholas Effect." Nicholas' own donation included heart, kidneys, liver, pancreas, and corneas. The seven recipients included four young people under age 20. In January, Reginald, Maggie, and Eleanor returned to Europe to receive the International Prize of Testimony from the Italian government.

Just recently, the Greens became the proud parents of twins. God does work in mysterious ways.

Besides the Greens and Patti Szuber, many equally special donors were honored at the ceremony for having given life's greatest gift. More than 40,300 (as of April 1995) Americans were on the waiting list for organ transplants at the time of this ceremony. In June 1996, more than 46,000 awaited the "gift of life." Now, more than 72,000 Americans are waiting for an organ transplant. On average, 16 people die each day in the United States because organs are not available.

Joesph Werling's wife, Peg, was 43 when she died of a stroke in January 1994. The family lived in West Chester, Ohio, in Greater Cincinnati. Peg was the mother of Nicole and Michelle Werling, and stepmother of Carrie, Stephanie, and Tracy Whittum. She was an organ and tissue donor. Werling owns his own company, Joe Werling Roofing and General Contracting. Carrie graduated from Miami University in Oxford, Ohio, in 1996; Stephanie graduated from Ohio State; Tracy, Nicole, and Michelle have also graduated or are still attending college.

Werling says Peg, who worked as a licensed practical nurse (LPN), was studying for her state boards to get her registered nurse (RN) license the night she had her stroke. "My wife was a nurse with the Veterans Administration Hospital in Cincinnati, and donating her organs and tissues would have made her very, very happy. A part of her lives on in others. Life was important to her and to give life to someone else was something she would have wanted."

Says Carrie of her stepmother: "It is very difficult to describe our mother (stepmother) without writing a book. She was the epitome of pure strength and love. While raising three girls, she worked full time as an LPN and put herself through school to become an RN. She always seemed to have time for her family and friends. She appreciated life and the people around her. There are so many wonderful gifts she left us, but the one that was most important was teaching us to love life and the people in it."

Donor families were welcomed to Washington, D.C., on Saturday evening, April 1, with a reception and program. On Sunday, they were honored guests at the National Donor Recognition Ceremony in the Great Hall of the Hubert H. Humphrey Building, U.S. Department of Health and Human Services. Assistant Surgeon General Dr. Kenneth P. Moritsuga, a donor husband, served as master of ceremonies. The event honored loved

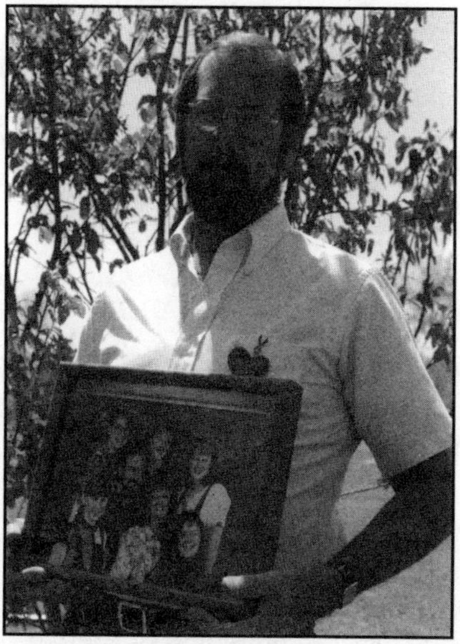

A Day to Remember

Joseph Werling spoke at a tree-planting ceremony on April 29, 1995, to honor Greater Cincinnati organ and tissue donors and their families. His wife, Peggy, was an organ and tissue donor in 1994.

Photograph © by Chris Cone

ones through music and remarks from donor families, transplant recipients and representatives of national transplant organizations.

"It meant so much to meet the recipients and their families," says Werling. "It was very emotional. I talked to one heart recipient for some time at the ceremony. When I was ready to leave, he asked me if it would be all right to give me a hug. At that time, I just broke down in tears. He was so grateful, as all recipients are, for their second chance. When we came back to the hotel from the ceremony, my 14-year-old daughter, Michelle, said as I was putting her to bed that she wanted to be a donor and have the sticker put on her driver's license when she turned 16."

Werling says he was honored to represent Cincinnati at the ceremony. Donor families received a letter from President Clinton for inclusion in a keepsake booklet. They also received a rosebud bouquet from the National Capital Area Chapter of Transplant Recipients International and a medallion in honor of their loved ones from the Central Pennsylvania Coalition on Donation. From Assistant Surgeon General Moritsuga, Werling received a certificate with the first names and last initials of all Greater Cincinnati organ donors in 1994. "I was very proud to have these," says Werling. The expanding Donor Family Quilt of the National Kidney Foundation was on display.

"We wish we could personally thank donor family members throughout the nation for each of their special gifts," said Judith Braslow, director of the DOT. "We hope that donor families who attended the ceremony will convey to other donor families in their localities our deepest appreciation for the lives they saved and improved."

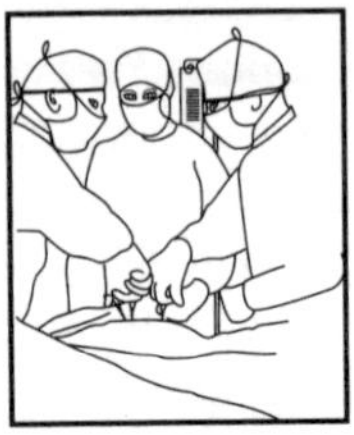

11

Pam Berkemeier: a beautiful young lady who gave life to others through death

Eighteen-year-old Pam Berkemeier died July 12, 1995, from injuries suffered in a single-car accident. The Edgewood, Kentucky, teenager had just graduated from Notre Dame Academy in Park Hills, Kentucky, and planned to attend Northern Kentucky State Vocational Technical School to study cosmetology. She was an organ and tissue donor.

Pam's parents, Roger and Ann Berkemeier, represented Cincinnati at the third annual National Donor Recognition Ceremony in Washington, D.C., on April 14, 1996. The ceremony, sponsored by the Division of Organ Transplantation (DOT), local organ and tissue procurement organizations, and transplant-related organizations, was held at the William H. Hatcher Conference Center on the campus of the National Institutes of Health. In 1995, more than three hundred people attended this ceremony. In 1996, about 450 donor family members, organ and tissue recipients, and their families attended. Among those who also attended were Senator Bill Frist (R-Tennessee), who is a heart transplant surgeon, and Jamie Redford, a liver recipient and son of actor/director Robert Redford. In Greater Cincinnati, LifeCenter and Ohio Valley Tissue and Skin Center sponsored the Berkemeiers.

The Berkemeiers appeared on WCPO-TV in Cincinnati after returning from the ceremony in Washington, D.C. Prior to the ceremony, the Berkemeiers were featured in a moving *Cincinnati Enquirer* editorial (Sunday, April 14, 1996) by deputy editor Linda Cagnetti. There was also a feature story on the Berkemeiers and Pam in the April 11, 1996, issue of the *Kenton County Recorder*, a northern Kentucky suburban newspaper. Finally, they were featured in a five-minute radio interview on WNKU, the radio station of Northern Kentucky University in Highland Heights, Kentucky. The interview won Associated Press public service awards in both Kentucky and Ohio for reporter Jay Hanselman and WNKU.

"Pam was always ready to accept everyone and listen or help if she could," says her mother, Ann. "She especially loved children and was a Big Sister during high school to a girl from the Kenton County Boys/Girls Club. Pam was a beautiful young lady who never saw herself that way. It was no surprise when she said she would like her organs and tissues donated if anything should happen to her. That is how she was, always thinking of someone else. I think it is fitting that one of her kidneys went to an 18-year-old girl who was looking forward to starting to college, just like Pam.

"From the day Pam was born, I always felt she was a very unique child. She was more mischievous than the other kids and nothing was out of her reach. In first grade, we found out she was dyslexic, and as a result she went for tutoring twice a week for seven years, including summers. Pam never complained about going and never missed school unless she was really sick.

"We can't understand why God took her, but we are thankful we had 18 wonderful years with her. Because of her love for others, there are several people who received organ and tissue transplants. We encourage everyone to give serious thought to organ and tissue donation. Many people can live a better life because of your love and thoughtfulness."

Pam's older sister, Lynne, a physical therapist at St. Elizabeth Medical Center South in northern Kentucky, says, "Pam's death brought intense grief and sorrow to many, many people, but especially her family. There is not a day that goes by that she is not the first thing I think about when I wake up and the last thing I think about before falling asleep. Thousands of things remind me of Pam; I am forever thinking of her. I have such an incredible sense of emptiness on the inside. The only remotely positive thing that came out of this whole nightmare is at least three people can lead a normal life because of Pam's donations. This is something Pam wanted. She talked to us about it after hearing a spokesperson from LifeCenter speak on the topic at school.

"Pam was a beautiful, caring 18-year-old girl who loved life, loved people, and loved the idea of being out of high school. She took in and cared for stray animals, and she knew her older sister better than anyone. All these things describe Pam. She fought for life for a week after her automobile accident July 5, 1995. It was so typical of her. She met every challenge head-on. She died July 12. Unfortunately, this was one problem I could not fix.

"None of us, Pam included, ever thought this would be something that would actually happen. Accidental deaths happen to other people, not my family (or so I thought). A tragic death did happen and my family was forced to make the decision about donating Pam's organs and tissues. Pam was the most giving person I know, so giving, even in her death, it seemed almost natural. There is some comfort in knowing that even in her death,

Pam lives on in others, both physically and spiritually. I encourage all families to discuss this difficult topic, even with young ones. As I've learned, death is not just for 'old' people, and organ and tissue donation can help others. And it offers some comfort to the remaining family members."

Pam's oldest brother, Steve, had this to say about his sister. "Pam was a caring and loving girl who faced all challenges head-on. She was a beautiful person who brought a smile to those around her, as her personality could light up a room. She was adventurous and unique in the ways she could touch our lives.

"Whether it was climbing the bookshelves before she could even walk, running around the house as a child covered in her mother's lipstick, showing her mashed potatoes as she ate them at the dinner table, or telling her leader at her senior retreat how much she loved and admired her older brother, Pam always managed to touch our hearts.

"She always thought of others first. Friends who were down or ill could count on Pam to be there to cheer them up. Pam was not only a great sister but a good friend. She was always fun to be around, whether it was at home or on vacation. One of my fondest memories of her is on one of our last vacations together. We took a long walk on the beach one morning and talked about everything. She was so neat. Not a day—not a minute—goes by where I don't think of her. I cherish the time I had with her but I'd give everything I have to get more time with her. She was one of a kind.

"Because Pam always thought of others, she had already stated her desire for organ and tissue donation. Here's a young kid thinking of others if the unforeseen should happen. Knowing that there was no hope for Pam's survival was the hardest thing I've ever been told in my life. The thought of her being gone was and is unbelievable. But she is not totally gone. Her spirit and memories live on through all of her family and friends. Others as well have lived on through Pam's desire for organ and tissue donation. It is the greatest gift anyone can give—life. I would encourage all to consider donation. Pam may be gone physically, but she lives on in my memories and in the organs and tissues she donated."

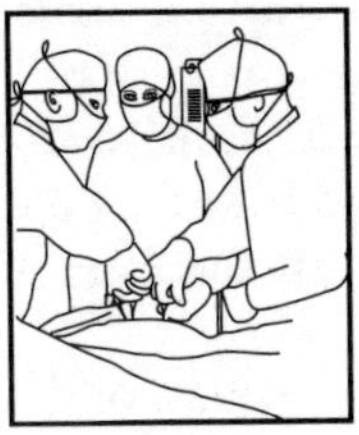

12

Janice Lail: a giving person who loved people

Forty-seven-year-old Janice Lail of Cincinnati died in May 1996. She was an organ and tissue donor. Her daughter, Marquita Barron, and mother, Ann Byrd, attended the fourth annual National Donor Recognition Ceremony and Workshop on Saturday and Sunday, April 12–13, 1997, at the Sheraton Washington Hotel in Washington, D.C. They were guests of LifeCenter. Barron and Byrd represented all 1996 organ and tissue donor families from Greater Cincinnati. Bryan Mills, formerly a transplant coordinator at LifeCenter, accompanied Barron and Byrd.

The ceremony was sponsored by the Division of Organ Transplantation (DOT). The National Donor Family Council of the National Kidney Foundation and other transplant organizations are also collaborators for this yearly event. LifeCenter and these organizations emphasize the importance of telling your family of your decision about organ and tissue donation.

The ceremony is a two-day event in the nation's capital paying tribute to all Americans who have donated their organs and tissues to save or improve the lives of others. It is also an opportunity for living donors and donor family members from across the country to share experiences, and remind the public of the continuing, urgent need for donors. The agenda of April 12 offered seminars and discussion groups on topics of interest to living donors and donor family members. The Sunday ceremony consisted of speakers and special tributes that focused on the generosity of America's silent heroes. Donor family members, living donors, transplant professionals, transplant recipients and the general public were invited. Acting Surgeon General Dr. Audrey F. Manley presented the surgeon general's Certificate of Appreciation to each donor family and living donor attending. David Crosby of Crosby, Stills, and Nash, and a November 1994 liver transplant recipient, attended the ceremony and was the key recipient speaker.

Lail worked in information systems at the Department of Health and Human Services. On a rainy May afternoon, she was going to Taft High

School to speak to students about career choices when she had to return to the building to get an umbrella. She suffered a ruptured aneurysm and fell on the steps. She died a short time later.

"When my grandmother (Ann Byrd) and I consented to donate my mother's organs and tissues, we based our decision on the way she structured her life," says Marquita Barron, Lail's daughter. "She was very religious and donation was something we knew she would want to do. Whenever someone needed something, and my mother had it, she would give it to them. The realization that she saved and improved the lives of others came after we received the donor family letter."

Byrd concurs saying, "We really didn't realize the importance of donation until after Janice's death. She was a giving person and loved people. I feel Janice's presence daily. When I saw her at the funeral home, she seemed to have a smile on her face. That lifted me up. She seemed to be saying, 'Thanks, mom, for donating my organs and tissues.'"

The 1997 program booklet included written tributes to donors whose families represented them at the ceremony or living donors who participated. The program also included a collage of living donors and donors whose families represented them at the ceremony. Donor families were also invited to contribute a quilt square in memory of their loved ones for the National Donor Family Quilt being created by the National Donor Family Council. Families may choose to place their donor's name, birthday, and date of death on the square. The National Donor Family Quilt is an ongoing endeavor.

Byrd spoke on behalf of organ and tissue donor families in Greater Cincinnati on April 27, 1997, at a tree-planting ceremony honoring 1996 donors and their families. It was held at Sharon Woods, a Hamilton County Park in Cincinnati.

"We who have donated saw something that needed to be done and we did it. I'm so proud to have represented you (donor families) in Washington, D.C. I found many aspects of the weekend special, especially recognizing a familiar pain in the eyes of others. I didn't ever feel uncomfortable to cry for I knew my new friends would understand the process of grief.

"Spending time with them in small group sessions, sharing the emotion and experience of the sudden and tragic loss of a loved one—fear, frustration, anger—they understood. Most importantly, they understood the tremendous value of organ and tissue donation and the grieving process. It was the beautiful act of giving that brought us together. I have slowly come to terms with the passing of Janice. But it is organ and tissue donation that has made a difference in how I see my Janice's death. I now understand that her end was someone else's beginning. She was always helping someone in some way. To be part of such a courageous and spiritual group reaffirmed that the decision we made to donate was the correct one."

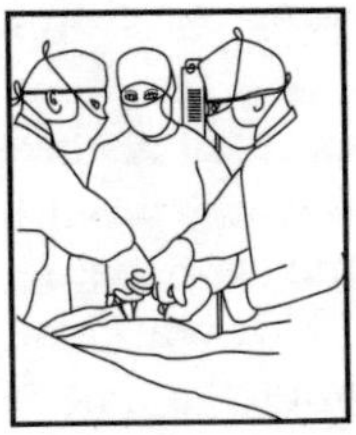

13

On the other side of the window

[*Author's Note: The following information was presented October 30, 1996, and November 4, 1998, during seminars called "Organ and Tissue Donation: Understanding the Process." Both were sponsored by LifeCenter. The presenter was Kathleen Doughman, RN, an in-patient critical care nurse at Bethesda North Hospital in Cincinnati. Kathleen's story was also published in the Summer 1997 issue of* UNOS Update); the *Fall 1997 issue of* LifeSource *(LifeCenter, Ohio Valley Tissue and Skin Center and the Cincinnati Eye Bank in Cincinnati); the September/October 1997 issue of* LifeLines *(Transplant Recipients International Organization); the January/February 1998 issue of* LifeLines *(Carolina LifeCare, Winston-Salem, North Carolina); the March 1998 issue of* Lifelines *(TransLife, Orlando, Florida); and the Summer 1998 issue of* OTAN *(American Red Cross, Lions Eye Bank of Nebraska and Nebraska Organ Retrieval System).*]

Some months ago, Wendy Valerius, a senior transplant coordinator with LifeCenter, came to our hospital to present a short in-service on organ and tissue donation. Following the in-service, as the nurses filtered out, I stayed behind, hoping to share with her a short story—one that I had hoped to share with someone from her organization for some time, actually for several years.

Wendy was kind and understanding. And I remember saying, "Wendy, I have thought about having an in-service of my own someday—being 'on the other side of the window.'" It was only a thought and I never dreamed I would have that opportunity.

I experienced a personal tragedy—an experience that changed my life and to this day causes me pain and a sense of great loss. That day, I made a decision, one that I am unable to take back. More times than I can count I have experienced a sense of remorse and guilt based on that decision. And I wonder, under the same circumstances, if you too may have made the same decision.

It was May 24, 1986, part of a beautiful Memorial Day weekend. I was planting flowers. It was my weekend off. It was my holiday off. Life was good! Suddenly, I glanced up from my planting to see a state highway patrol cruiser coming down my driveway. I immediately thought of my son, Terry. Had he been speeding? Could there have been an accident? He had been out of high school for a year and I knew he had fallen in with the wrong crowd. I had suspicions he was experimenting with drugs. When I would ask, he would always say, "Mom, you worry too much, everything is fine!"

I noticed at times he had mood swings, but when you have three teenagers, sometimes those are to be expected. At times he did cause disruptions in our home. Friends or family members would tell me now that he was out of school, maybe I should tell him to find a place of his own. "You shouldn't have to put up with all that aggravation," they would say. But I loved him. I did not care for his friends and I thought if I am the only positive influence in his life, then he can stay at home as long as he wants. He was my firstborn. I had him when I was 19. I had him for half of my life. I prayed for him every day. I did not think anything could happen to anyone you loved so much and prayed for every day. I was wrong.

The state highway patrolman got out of his car, took off his hat, and said, "Mrs. Doughman, is your husband here? Your son has been shot and you need to get to a certain hospital immediately. I wiped my soiled hands on my pants and my husband and I got into the car and rushed to the hospital.

Time does not permit me to tell you the thoughts and events of that journey. It was one of the longest in my life.

When we arrived at the hospital, for the first time I was on "the other side of the window." I tapped on the glass window, identified myself, and asked if I could please speak with the nurse caring for my son. I felt helpless, frightened and alone.

We were ushered to a small room adjacent to the nurses' station. The nurse looked me in the eyes and said, "Your son is brain dead. He is on a ventilator. Would you like to donate any organs?" One sentence, without taking a breath, is how I found out that my son was dead.

Later I was to learn from my pastor that Terry was very remorseful about using drugs and he felt he had gotten himself into something he could not get out of. Teenagers are very impulsive. There is no tomorrow or next month for them. They think in the here and now. Terry died of a self-inflicted gunshot wound to the head. He went to a quiet pond where he liked to go fishing and took his own life rather than go back on substances that had begun to rob him of his will, his self-esteem, and good judgment. I lost a beautiful, sensitive child that day. I lost part of myself that day also.

Weeks before the first anniversary date of my son's death, I was truly starting to fall apart. I could not stand to think of facing his birthday, May 21, and the day of his death, May 24—two significant dreaded anniversary dates in the same week! I was panicking and in tremendous pain. I believe, not by chance, but as a "gift to me in my grief," I met another nurse in our hospital, Alice Weening, with whom I now work. She lost her 13-year-old son, Kevin, three and a half weeks after I lost Terry. She told me about a support group for bereaved parents called Compassionate Friends.

Up until that time I had thought very little about organ donation or the decision I had made the previous year. I was consumed in my own grief. I attended the Compassionate Friends meeting that month and continued to attend the monthly meetings.

There are times as we go around the circle that a parent will pull out a folded letter and with tears streaming down their faces, say, "My son's heart went to a 26-year-old father. He has a little girl three years old." Or "My daughter's liver went to a 52-year-old gentleman with children and grandchildren. They say he is doing wonderfully."

And the parents hold these letters close to their hearts. They are so thankful, knowing that a part of their child lives on. And this feeling provides them with a measure of comfort. I have no letter. No part of my son lives on, sparing another family the excruciating pain of loss. I made a decision that day when I was "on the other side of the window."

I cannot begin to impress upon you as healthcare professionals, the impact your words have on these family members. They may forget your name or your face, but they will never forget those words informing them that their loved one has expired and the manner in which you request an anatomical gift. For years, each month at our Compassionate Friends meetings, as a legacy to our sons, Alice and I counsel the most newly bereaved, trying to provide them with a measure of hope. In time the pain will subside, and yes, in time, life will take on meaning once again. Many of these dear parents paid the ultimate sacrifice to help another human being.

Many years ago I felt I was done a great injustice by one of my peers. I have been a nurse all my life. I began as a candy striper at age 15. I would never have been so insensitive to a family member at the time of their loss.

I would ask you to be sensitive as you inquire about an anatomical gift. Be sensitive to a family who loved, shared a history with, or, as in my case, brought this patient into the world. It is a painful time. It is a difficult decision. And please remember that your words and deeds are never forgotten.

With all the recent hospital politics and cutbacks, I think we have all lost a little heart and perhaps have forgotten the reason we chose this profession. But the cutbacks and politics are not the fault of the patient or family.

Had I been approached differently, I, too, may have been a donor family member. What decision would you have made if it were your child?

It is my prayer that if you ever find yourself "on the other side of the window" that you are met with sincere kindness and compassion. For:

Sometimes love is for a moment,
Sometimes love is for a lifetime,
Sometimes a moment is a lifetime.

Section III

Transplant Friends and Other Recipient Stories

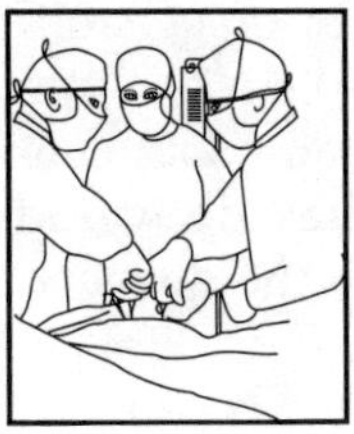

14

Patty Britton: strengthened by faith, family, and friends

Since my heart transplant in 1989, I have met many wonderful people who have gone through an organ transplant. At first, it was just heart transplant recipients when I joined the cardiac transplant support group, Change of Heart, at University Hospital in Cincinnati. But I have also met and made friends with others who have liver, kidney, and kidney/pancreas transplants. I think we are all special people who exhibit courage, faith, and yes, even fear sometimes. We value this second chance we have been granted and try to help each other. God guides us in our everyday lives. We live with the knowledge that someone we never knew or met has saved our lives. It is a rewarding feeling that humbles us each time we look in the mirror, and with every breath and step we take.

In this section are just a few of my many transplant friends. There are many, many more. I know you'll enjoy reading about them.

* * * * *

In the fall of 1994, Paul and Patty Britton were looking forward to the birth of their first child. But Patty had to go into the hospital, St. Elizabeth Medical Center South, in Edgewood, Kentucky, on November 28, 1994. She needed complete bed rest to treat preeclampsia, a toxic condition developing in late pregnancy characterized by a sudden rise in blood pressure, excessive weight gain, edema, albuminuria, severe headache, and visual disturbances. "I was there for two weeks and then one night something went wrong," remembers Patty vividly. "I was in terrible, terrible pain."

Paul and Patty live in Hebron, Kentucky. Both graduated from the University of Nebraska in the late 1980s. They both met there as students. Paul is from New Jersey. Patty is from Fairfield, Nebraska, a small farming community. In 1989, they moved to New Jersey where Paul took a job as an operations manager for a steel company. In 1991, he went to work for another steel company, International Mold Steel, and they moved to Houston. International Mold Steel moved to Erlanger, Kentucky, and in

September 1993 the Brittons moved to Hebron. Patty took a job as an administrative assistant at CBS Personnel in Cincinnati. "We have been here ever since," says Paul.

The preeclampsia began when Patty was seven months' pregnant and went in for her monthly obstetrician appointment. "We had just had Paul's family for Thanksgiving," says Patty. "I had been in the hospital since November 28. The night of December 10, I was having severe pains. I remember screaming in my room at the hospital and then they delivered Christopher by emergency cesarean section. Usually, with the delivery, preeclampsia turns itself around." The doctors at St. Elizabeth thought the severe pain was the point when Patty's liver died or clotted because of disseminating intravascular coagulation (DIC), a condition which clots off an organ and usually settles in that organ. "The doctors thought it settled in my liver."

Patty's problems were not over yet. She was a very, very sick young woman. Finally, on December 17, Patty was transferred to University Hospital in Cincinnati and put under the care of Dr. Douglas Hanto, director of the liver transplant program and professor of surgery. "At that point," says Patty, "Dr. Hanto had three options: Wait another 24 hours to see if I would turn the corner; do a piggyback liver transplant; or do a liver transplant. And I didn't know any of this because I was in a coma by then. I guess when Dr. Hanto and his team opened me up, they knew I needed a liver transplant." According to Paul, Patty got the transplant within eight hours. Patty probably had only 24 hours to live. "I had the transplant December 17 and I didn't come out of the coma until December 23." Patty lost her first liver transplant, not because of rejection, but because the liver acted as a sponge for the DIC. It was an extra large liver and Dr. Hanto thought about cutting it down because it was so big. The DIC took 75 percent of it. Patty had her second liver transplant February 11 and was in University Hospital until she was transferred to Drake Center in Cincinnati, a long-term care and rehabilitation hospital.

For Patty's entire hospitalization and rehabilitation—St. Elizabeth Medical Center South, University Hospital and Drake Center—her mother, Joyce Schlick, was with her and Paul. A retired school nurse who now serves as a summer camp nurse in Fairfield, a small, rural Nebraska farming community, Joyce stayed with Patty and Paul in Hebron until Mother's Day 1995. "Mom does not work full time," says Patty. "And she enjoys her opportunities to travel and go at will." Patty's father died in 1993. Her grandfather, Joyce's father, died while Patty was in a coma.

Dr. Hanto and Dr. John Valente, then a liver transplant fellow at University Hospital (now a transplant surgeon in Portland, Oregon) allowed Joyce to sleep in the empty bed next to Patty in her room during her hospitalization. "As a nurse, she knew what was going on and maybe some of the time she did not want to know," says Paul.

"When other people did not know if my condition was bad or good, she knew right away," interjects Patty.

"It was a double-edged sword for Joyce," continues Paul. "Sometimes a little knowledge is a dangerous thing. Dr. Hanto and Dr. Valente knew when they blocked off the room for Joyce what she would do for Patty. Between her first and second liver transplant, Patty was very sick. Food did not stay down. Patty could not get up or get out of bed herself. With Joyce there, everything got done."

"I was developing an ulcer and was given Prilosec® to make my stomach contract so food could pass through easier. I threw up constantly while I was in the hospital. It was funny because Paul would go out to get he and Mom something to eat and they'd be sitting there in my room with me throwing up, and they would just hand me an emesis pan and keep eating at the same time. We laughed a lot too. It was a terrible situation, but you had to laugh and make the best of it.

"I had 24-hour care. The nurse had 10 to 12 other patients. University Hospital was going through a phase of cutting the nursing staffs. I felt bad for these nurses because they would come into my room and they were just frazzled. It was a saving grace that Mom was there. She would pick up on things that maybe the nurses who came in only once in a while wouldn't pick up on." The nurses did not have to stop at Patty's room unless there was a problem. "They also enjoyed talking to my mom. And they had her right there if they needed help."

There was one time in University Hospital when Patty was having problems breathing. Dr. Hanto came in one morning on rounds and Mom said, "I do not know what it is, but I'm seeing this, this, and this, and I don't like what I'm seeing." Within 10 minutes they were tapping Patty's lungs to draw fluid.

Another time, right after Patty was out of surgery, she had a problem with gastrointestinal bleeding that they had just stopped. "I was given K-exylate® to lower the potassium level in my blood," she says. "It lowered my potassium but started the gastrointestinal bleeding again. Dr. Hanto canceled that order almost immediately.

"There were various things that happened and Mom knew enough to question them. I'm not saying the staff or residents were bad, but there were times when she saved me from major mistakes. The nurses would come in my room in the morning, look at my chart on the wall, and ask Mom for a rundown. They liked that, although there was some question as to who my primary nurse was. Mom was careful not to overstep her bounds."

While hospitalized, Patty would occasionally have student nurses taking care of her. "The student nurse director invited Mom to one of her classes to speak," relates Patty.

Patty and Paul are quick to admit that Dr. Hanto and Dr. Valente were the best team they have ever seen. And they both credit the staff at St. Elizabeth Medical Center South with keeping Patty alive prior to her two transplants.

Patty does not know too much about her donors. The first donor was a large male from Toledo, Ohio. The second one was a young man, 28, who was Patty's height and weight. He died of a brain aneurysm. "The residents would come into my room on rounds before the second transplant," says Patty. She'd ask if they had a liver for her yet. And they'd say they had a few calls. "I was just so amazed at how much information they knew about potential donors. And they always kept saying, 'We want the perfect liver. We're not going to settle for second best.'"

In the meantime, Christopher was in the neonatal intensive care unit (NICU) at Children's Hospital Medical Center (CHMC) in Cincinnati. "When he was born," recalls Patty, "they basically told Paul they didn't think he would make it since he was premature. Amazingly so, he did. He was at St. Elizabeth and then stabilized and transferred to CHMC."

While she was still in University Hospital, Patty did get to see Christopher. It was a traumatic experience for her. She had just undergone an emergency C-section and two liver transplants, did not know if she would make it, and knew that Christopher might not make it either. "It was a surreal situation," remembers Patty. "I can still remember waking up from my coma, but I don't remember anything from the night I was in such severe pain and had Christopher. I don't remember anything from then until I woke up after my first liver transplant. I remember hearing my mom's voice and she said, 'Patty, you're at University Hospital. You had a baby boy, Christopher, and he's over at Children's. He's doing OK.' Then she said, 'You've had a liver transplant.' And I couldn't speak because of the respirator, but I can just remember (thinking), What? I had what? The last thing I remember was being pregnant in St. Elizabeth's. I don't know, it was hard to be going to see Christopher because I had not seen him since he was born.

"It was funny visiting him because they wheeled me over to CHMC with my IV stand and they had me all bundled up. It was late February 1995. I was in a wheelchair because I was so debilitated I could not even roll over in bed. I could not lift my arms. I could not stand by myself. They took me through the tunnels at University Hospital and across the street to CHMC. Paul, a resident, two nurses and my mom were with me. I had on a surgical mask and a blanket over my head as they were wheeling me across the street! I thought, this is really ridiculous. But I did get to hold Christopher. It was strange. It did not seem like he was mine. It was really hard being separated."

Patty says the neonatal staff at CHMC was always hopeful and very positive regarding Christopher's condition. Dr. James M. Greenberg, head of the neonatal intensive care unit (NICU) at CHMC, "was a wonderful man. He came over to see me in the surgical intensive care unit (SICU) at University Hospital. He said, 'You know, I'm Christopher's doctor and it is not the greatest...but we have hope for him.' Dr. Greenberg and his nurses came to see me personally to give me updates. The nurses took lots of pictures and posted them in my room. I have a few pictures of him. Towards the end, it was kind of like a contest. I had to get better so I could beat Christopher out of the hospital."

Paul says the ordeal with Patty and Christopher was "pure hell, plain and simple, for both of them. I was never more helpless in my life. It is something I do not ever want to go through again. It was just terrible." Though Paul and Patty had the support of their families, they say the pain did not go away. Paul has two brothers and two sisters. Patty has one brother who lives in Fairfield, Nebraska, and runs a 1,300-acre farm. He is married and has three children.

"They all flocked in at a moment's notice," recalls Patty. "Our moms were here first and then the rest of the families started coming in. We were very lucky. Our families are very close even though they are miles apart."

Christopher was in the NICU at CHMC from December 10, 1994, until he died March 30, 1995. Paul and Patty felt as if Christopher had a mission—to make sure that Patty was going to be okay. Patty was released from University Hospital February 28, 1995. "It was like he knew I was home and that I was going to be OK, and that his mission on earth was done and he could go now."

Paul and Patty donated Christopher's corneas for transplant. "We got a letter from the Cincinnati Eye Bank thanking us for our donation," says Paul. "It was tough. There wasn't really much the doctors could do for Christopher at CHMC."

Patty agrees, saying, "He was sick for so long. The DIC had infected his lungs. We were at Children's Hospital the night Christopher died. We were prepared to spend the night. I had been given two wonderful gifts of life. I was almost disappointed we could not do more. It was kind of interesting to us, being on both sides, transplantation and donation. You definitely have a different perspective and it was very fresh for us."

Christopher was buried in Patty's small Nebraska hometown, Fairfield. Fairfield has a population of about five hundred people. Patty's grandparents and her dad are buried there. "We didn't really know what to do because we had only been in Hebron for two years."

After Patty's release from University Hospital, she entered Drake Center in Cincinnati for physical rehabilitation. She was at Drake from March 3 until March 27. Patty says her experience at University Hospital and at Drake was a weird feeling. "You are living a normal life and then all of a sudden you realize you've got somebody else's liver inside your body keeping you alive. I was in a wheelchair. I could not walk. Rehabilitation was hard because I really was debilitated, especially my abdominal muscles and back. When they transferred me to University Hospital from St. Elizabeth for the liver transplant, I weighed 220 pounds. My kidneys had shut down and I was full of fluid. Dr. Hanto was concerned about my therapy and he really wanted me to get more but since there was not much time between my first and second transplant, I got a little better but not much better. I just didn't have any energy. They did as much as they could at University Hospital and then transferred me to Drake, a little less than a month after my second transplant."

Patty says the idea was not just to get her into physical therapy, work with her and get done. "It was a very humbling experience, having to learn to walk all over. I'm a very independent person, always have been, and to have to rely on people so much for everything—to roll over in bed, go to the bathroom, brush my teeth, to do everything because I could hardly lift my arms—was very frustrating."

But Patty also realized at Drake that she would walk again and be herself. "I saw around me people who would never have the chance to walk again," she says sadly.

After her release from Drake Center, Patty still had a long way to go. She was still in a wheelchair and could not walk by herself. She entered a physical therapy program at St. Elizabeth Medical Center South, working three to four days a week for an hour at a time with physical therapist Lynne Berkemeier. Patty was in this program from the end of March 1995 until June 1995. "She was great," says Patty of Lynne. "She had never dealt with a transplant patient before. She was so good because she would push me to do a little bit more. I'd get tired and she'd say, 'Are you in pain or just tired?' She was very positive and we laughed a lot. But it was intensive. I'd get my lab work done at St. Elizabeth and go to physical therapy. Mom went with me. She was part of my therapy too. She made sure I did not just stay in the house. She dragged me all over the place."

Lynne had a very positive effect on Patty. At the end of Patty's therapy, Lynne gave her a book, *The Little Engine That Could.* "I still have it," says Patty. "Lynne and I keep in touch." Sadly, Lynne's younger sister, Pam, died in a single car accident July 12, 1995. Pam was an organ and tissue donor. Lynne's parents, Roger and Ann, of Edgewood, Kentucky, attended the National Donor Recognition Ceremony in Washington, D.C., April 14, 1996. (See chapter 11).

When Patty's physical therapy ended in June, she still had to use a walker. "I had to learn how to drive a car again," she says. "I was afraid to drive. I didn't know how quick my reactions would be. So we went to Florence Mall near our house. I got in the car, and fortunately, it was no big deal. And I drove home. But it was scary at first. I was learning everything all over again."

Paul interjects it is not really mental learning, but muscular learning. "Your mind can do it, but your body doesn't react to (driving) as well. I wanted her to speed up and stop quickly to see if her reaction time was OK. The test was to see if her muscles could do it."

Around Thanksgiving 1996, Patty began experiencing some serious problems. Her hepatic artery became clogged. She developed a cyst on her liver. On March 28, 1997, Patty had her third liver transplant at University Hospital with the same surgical team. Her prognosis is good.

Today, Patty enjoys walking. "My stamina is almost completely back," she says. "I used to do aerobics at the gym for an hour. Now I exercise 30 to 50 minutes three to four times a week. After three liver transplants and a C-section, I have few stomach muscles left. It takes a long time to build them back. We belong to a fitness center now in Edgewood, Kentucky."

As for follow-up care, Patty gets periodic lab work. She takes several immunosuppressive drugs to prevent rejection, cyclosporine, azathioprine, and prednisone. She is also on a diuretic, antibiotic, Prilosec®, and multivitamins.

Patty takes her medication on time and every day. "I don't even think there is a choice," she says bluntly. "Paul often tells me I'm more aware of my health than most normal people. I take my blood pressure nightly and temperature daily. Being more aware of my health keeps me healthier. It is not just a choice."

The outpouring of support from friends, neighbors, hospital staff and co-workers makes Paul and Patty feel very grateful. CBS Personnel had a "Spirit of Patty Britton Drive" in which they sold sweatshirts with the CBS logo and donated the proceeds to the Brittons. CBS also took up collections on "casual days" to help defray medical costs. Get-well cards and groceries came from neighbors and co-workers. The nurses at University Hospital threw Patty a baby shower. "My belief in human kindness was greatly reinforced, sometimes by people I didn't even know," she says.

Patty and Christopher's hospital and doctor bills were enormous. In the spring of 1996, Patty called her health insurance case manager. "Carrie, I said," recalls Patty, "do you know how much our bills are? I think it was $549,000 for just me. With Christopher's bills it was much higher." This does not include the cost of Patty's third liver transplant. "Paul and I need to evaluate our insurance because I only have $1 million lifetime coverage. But CIGNA® was just great. We didn't have any problems at all."

The liver transplant program at University Hospital recently formed a support group, thanks in part to Patty. "I've also helped develop a pre-transplant and post-transplant brochure for patients who come to clinic." There is also a telephone tree for the transplant office for those patients interested in support but who may not be able to make it to meetings. "We

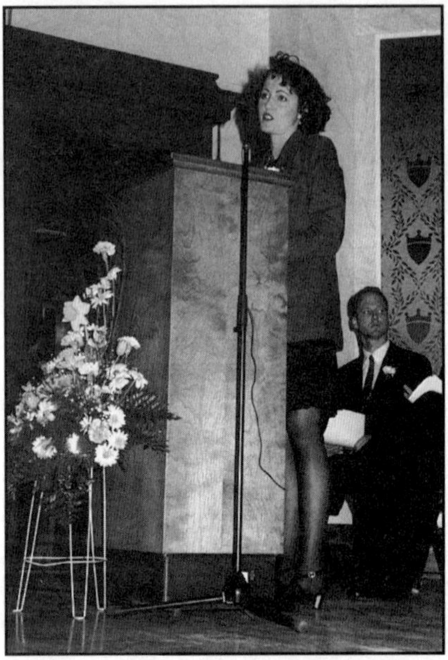

A Recipient's Story

Patty Britton, a liver transplant recipient and donor mother, shares her poignant story of triumph over tragedy at a Donor Family Ceremony at Cincinnati's Memorial Hall on April 19, 1998.

Photograph © by Art Badger

want it to be not only an emotional support group, but educational and social too. Those are our three goals and objectives."

Reflecting on her whole ordeal, Patty's philosophy is simple: "There was a reason I was spared and am still around. I could have very easily died. Maybe the reason is to get the word out about organ and tissue donation. I feel strongly about promoting it. I like talking to people about organ and tissue donation. I find the different views of people interesting. With Christopher gone, maybe God has some babies out there who might not have a chance at life and Paul and I are here to provide them better lives. My faith has grown stronger. Learning about how the body works, how intricate things are, you have to believe in a higher being. No mortal man could create the human body. The advances man has made and the knowledge we have about the human body are incredible, especially when you are talking about transplantation."

Patty sent thank-you letters to all three of her donor families. "There are not enough words to express my gratitude," she says tearfully. "I told them a little bit about me. I wanted them to know my liver disease was not because I abused my body. The doctors said it was because I was so healthy and in good condition that I pulled through. I was pregnant but I exercised and took care of myself and continue to do so. I let them know we lost Christopher but we did donate his corneas. I wanted to let them know we are going to adopt children. I think it would give them good feelings or some peace to know they helped me and I went on to help somebody else. All donor families are recognized as heroic. I still think they are incredible people for the decisions they have made. I know those decisions were very hard."

Today, after her third liver transplant, Patty is a founding board member of the Tri-State Liver Transplant Support Group at University Hospital and edits its newsletter, *The Liver Times*. She still works for CBS Personnel

Services in Cincinnati and is a certified volunteer with LifeCenter, helping promote organ and tissue donation to the public. She and Paul recently adopted a baby, Nicholas William.

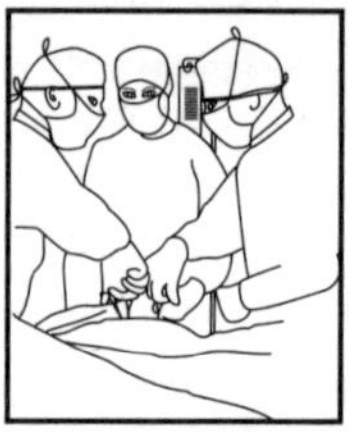

15

Jack Stranko's faith, family, and positive attitude play key roles in his health

Jack Stranko is a man of great faith. In April 1976, he suffered a severe heart attack in the airport at LaCrosse, Wisconsin. He was on a business trip. "I always thought that I was going to make it through," he says. "I just went over and stood in front of the fan as I was waiting for my plane. I didn't tell anybody. I didn't go to the hospital. I was waiting for a late plane and I wanted to get home. And I just sat there and it was hurting and hurting and I was just praying and praying it would stop. After about 15 to 20 minutes the pain stopped. And I knew it was a heart attack because my father had heart problems."

Between April and September 1976, Stranko had four more heart attacks. "The heart attacks I experienced were all very painful," admits Stranko. "The pain would start in the center of my chest and go over to my left shoulder and down my left arm to my elbow. And it literally felt like a dump truck was sitting on that part of my body. In those days, they wanted you to wait six weeks before getting an arteriogram after a heart attack. But every time six weeks would roll around I'd have another heart attack. Finally, by the end of the summer, I had one at University Hospital." His cardiologist was Dr. John Holmes. He said Stranko needed bypass surgery. Stranko was sent to the Texas Heart Institute in Houston. Renowned heart transplant surgeon Dr. Denton Cooley, a pioneer in cardiac transplant, did his bypass surgery. "I thought I was going down there for three bypasses and he came in and talked to me one evening and said, 'No, Jack, I think I'll just give you five.'"

Cooley told Stranko after the surgery, "I would have given you six but you had one artery that was completely stopped up during one of the heart attacks and that part of your heart died."

This was in October 1976. "I'll do them now and then I won't have to worry about you for 10 years. I won't have to see you for 10 years." Stranko was 45 years old at the time. Stranko recently corresponded with Dr. Cooley.

"And he was right," admits Stranko. Prior to my heart transplant I had one more heart attack in 1984. With that one, my heart just started deteriorating. And then two years later I had the transplant."

Stranko looked tired and emaciated before the transplant. Newspaper photos attest to his appearance. He saw Dr. Raymond Timmerman, his family doctor in January 1986. "He put his finger on it," says Stranko, "saying I needed a heart transplant. I had lost about 45 pounds in three months. I had become jaundiced because I wasn't pumping any blood through my heart. It was pumping at about 10 percent. I looked terrible." Dr. Holmes verified Stranko's need of a heart transplant when Stranko entered St. Luke Hospital East in Fort Thomas, Kentucky, in late January 1986. Stranko had not seen Dr. Holmes since his bypass surgery 10 years earlier.

"I sat on the side of the bed all that night, thinking about having a heart transplant," says Stranko. "My wife, Peggy, never knew about this. Everyone was gone when they told me this. I was all by myself in that room and I just kept praying all night. When my son came up to my room the next morning, I was still sitting on the side of the bed and I thought *I'm going to do this thing. I'm going to get this transplant because I don't want to be a burden to anybody the rest of my life. If there's any way I can get up and get moving on my own rather than have somebody take care of me the rest of my life I'll do it.*

The next day, at St. Luke's, Stranko met Dr. David Melvin who ran the heart transplant program at University Hospital. Prior to this, Stranko only knew that on December 17, 1985, Charlie Ashcraft of Cold Spring, Kentucky, became the first heart transplant recipient at University Hospital. "I saw Charlie on TV at Christmas time," says Stranko. "And I looked at him and I was losing weight and didn't know where I was headed. I commented to Peggy, 'Look at him. He had a heart transplant two weeks ago and he's going home!'

"I couldn't believe it. I didn't know Charlie personally, but I was just amazed at him going home and looking good! Little did I know that four months later I'd be going home with one. That's all I knew about transplants."

Dr. Melvin came to see Jack about 10 or 11 A.M. He introduced himself. "The first thing I said to Dr. Melvin," recalls Stranko, "and he looked like the kind of guy you could just pour your heart out to, right from the beginning, like you wouldn't have any trouble at all talking to him was, 'Dr. Melvin, do you believe in divine healing?' And he looked at me and said, 'Yes, I do Jack. I'm a born-again Christian and I'm here doing the Lord's work.' When I heard that I said that's all I needed to know. I said let's get on with this thing. That's how we met."

For the next several months, Dr. Melvin and the cardiac transplant team at University Hospital evaluated Stranko. He spent two weeks in Holmes Hospital (affiliated with the University Hospital) for tests. His final tests before being put on the waiting list for a new heart were in early April 1986. Dr. Melvin told Stranko it would probably be a four- to six-week wait for a heart. The last cardiac test he had was an angiogram. It was on April 11. He had the test at University Hospital and then went home. Later that evening a heart became available from Cleveland. Stranko was transplanted on April 12, 1986, the eighth heart transplant recipient in Cincinnati.

After he was transplanted and out of the cardiac intensive care unit, he was put in a specially ventilated room. Peggy came in to see him. She noticed in the room next to him was a man named Luebbe, but she didn't stop. "I was awake then," recalls Stranko.

She said, "There's a man over there whose name is Luebbe. I wonder if that's Ed Luebbe?" Ed was her childhood sweetheart. "I'm going to walk over and see if he's the same Ed Luebbe." So she walked over and sure enough it was him.

"I was number eight and he was number nine," says Stranko. "He was her childhood sweetheart and I ended up marrying her."

Stranko still keeps in contact with Dr. Melvin. He tells an interesting anecdote about the dedication and sincerity of Dr. Melvin. Cardiac transplant recipients require frequent heart biopsies to detect rejection.

"Dr. Melvin was a hardworking man," says Stranko. "He lived in that hospital. You know all doctors have problems. I thought the world of him and I still do. I was in there for a biopsy one time close to Christmas and something was wrong and he was fiddling around and could not get the bioptome to go down into my jugular vein."

"Jack, I've fiddled with you long enough. I don't want to put you through any more. Let's knock it off and come back next week and we'll try it again."

"I was the first patient that morning. And I thought, boy, I'm going to destroy his day. So I asked him about going in the other side?"

He said, "Do you want to try that? Are you willing to try that?"

"So he went in under the clavicle and we got the thing over with. And I know he felt good about it and so did I. And you know he sent me a Christmas card and he told me I was a blessing to him. You know, **he** tells **me** that I'm a blessing to him! He doesn't know the blessing he was to me."

Stranko is a very good Christian. He is a Cathacostal, attending both a Pentacostal church and St. Thomas More Catholic Church in Amelia, Ohio. He also sings and plays the guitar in the choirs of these churches. Dr. Melvin invited him to make the walk to Emmanas at the United Methodist Church in Hyde Park, a Cincinnati suburb. In fact, Dr. Melvin sponsored him and then had to go to Austria for a two-year course of study in mechanical heart assist devices. "He felt bad about having sponsored me and then having to leave," recalls Stranko. "It was a big deal. On the last night when you come out of this dark room you walk up this long, winding stairway and then the person who sponsors you usually meets you and walks down through the church with you. But he couldn't be there, so I didn't know what was going to happen. He sent his son, who I also knew. I almost cried because he thought enough to think about having somebody there for me."

Besides his wife, Peggy, Stranko has been blessed with four children and nine grandchildren. All live within a stone's throw of him and Peggy.

"I had all the support anyone could ask for," says Stranko. "They never questioned whether I should or shouldn't have the transplant. My daughter Melinda (Mindy) said she was going to talk to me a couple of times when I was going through this sick period before the transplant. She wanted me to consider a transplant. She didn't even know I was going to have one. There were many times during that 10-year period in my life when despair could have gripped the hearts and minds of those close to me. But encouragement and support were all that my family demonstrated. I thank them for having the faith and strength necessary to stay on an even keel and for not wavering in their resolve that all would be well in spite of what was going on around me. Still, through it all, I worked all the way up until the time I went into the hospital for the transplant."

Stranko worked at Ellis and Watts in Cincinnati for 40 years. He was in the Air Force from 1948 until 1954. He knew General Chuck Yeager, one of the Air Force's first test pilots, when he was stationed at Edwards Air Force base in California. Said good morning to him each day. Ellis and Watts manufactures custom-made cooling equipment for the electronics, aerospace and nuclear industry. Their equipment has been on space shots and communication shelters. They also manufactured mobile trailers to hold MRI and CT scanners. Stranko built the first mobile CT system in Europe with General Electric.

Stranko started off with the drafting and design group at Ellis and Watts and worked there for 12 years before moving into manufacturing. "I got associated with every facet of the business—from design to engineering to purchasing and quality control. I ended up being the manufacturing manager. We had a work force of over 250. I ran the plant for many years." In 1996, he retired from Ellis and Watts.

Stranko attributes his heart problems to poor eating habits, not exercising, and smoking, and says that as much as 50 percent could have been hereditary. He smoked about a pack of cigarettes a day.

"Smoking is a terrible habit, an addiction," he says. "It's as bad as any drug ever was. I have a hard time jumping on anybody because they don't quit smoking. I always recommend they quit and tell them not to smoke, and pray for them, but I have a hard time getting tough with them because I know what a problem it was for me to quit smoking."

Stranko was so addicted in fact, that he craved a cigarette on the way home from the hospital after his transplant. He smoked from 1979 until his transplant in 1986. "I smoked right up until the time I went into the hospital to get the transplant! I didn't smoke for the two weeks I was in the hospital. On my way home from the hospital, I told my wife I wanted to stop and get a pack of cigarettes. You talk about a sick person! That's how much of a hold those cigarettes had on me. We got in a real argument over it. She said she wouldn't stop. I said when I get home I'll just walk down to the corner and buy a pack. Well, I finally came to my senses when I saw how bad it hurt her and my oldest daughter, Kathy, who was with us. They both started crying and I never picked up another cigarette. Never have to this day. But I wanted that cigarette the day I came out of the hospital."

Stranko not only has a great deal of faith, but also practices positive thinking. Following is an excerpt from the Change of Heart support group newsletter (March 1995) from University Hospital. He is speaking for all heart recipients here.

> *FEAR is the biggest single obstacle we have to overcome. This FEAR keeps us from living a normal, productive life after having a transplant. This FEAR is our enemy, and that is the way we have to think of it. It is always present in our mind, waiting to pounce on every emotional experience we may encounter. That is if we let it fester inside us.*
>
> *Am I saying that I never experienced FEAR? No, I'm not saying that, because I would be lying if I said that FEAR is not a normal reaction for everyone, before and after transplant.*
>
> *The BEFORE FEAR disappears for most of us within a few weeks following surgery, when once again we are able to think clearly and we realize we made it through the most difficult part. Physically we may still be on a low, but mentally we are on a high.*
>
> *For most of us, this high is short-lived because now come the AFTER FEARS, the two words, biopsy and rejection. Two words we heard about before the transplant, but paid little attention to are now real and we (heart transplant recipients) have to learn to deal with them for the rest of our lives. Unlike the BEFORE FEARS, an operation won't make these AFTER FEARS go away.*
>
> *For lack of a better word, these two 'necessary evils' are at the bottom of most NEGATIVE ATTITUDES. Think about it. If it wasn't for our fear of having a biopsy and the possibility of rejection, along with all the special drugs, the costs and the required check-ups, this transplant stuff would be a piece of cake!*
>
> *That is not the way it is though, and it looks like we are stuck with all these things. So why not try to make the best of it and stop making yourself and everyone around you miserable with a poor attitude. You must change your way of thinking because that is where it all starts.*
>
> *First you have to realize how blessed you are. I do not believe some of us ever give it a second thought. Do not put it off; think about it, you are a*

blessed person! You are one of a very unique group of people. You have been given a second shot at being able to live a 'quality life.' Don't waste it on negative thinking, worry and fear. The donor did their part, and now it's up to you to do your part. Your attitude is the most important part.

I could talk forever about the rewards of having a positive attitude, but I think I'll get right to the point and share with you what I believe and why it works for me.

First, I have a strong belief and faith in the miracle-working power of God.

Second, when I have a serious concern of any kind, in any area of my life, not just with my heart, God is the first one I turn to for help.

Third, if it's a condition I can do something about, I do all that is within my power, because that is doing my part. If it is a condition that I can do nothing about, and I have no control over it, I immediately give the problem to God so He can do his part. After all, He is the only one who can find a way when there is no way.

Here is how I put this faith, which removes all my FEAR and is the driving force behind my positive attitude, into action. I tell you this not to be boasting, but only so you will know exactly how I use this gift to help me in time of need.

I'll use my preparation for a biopsy as an example, since this is a common concern we all share. This is how I start preparing and this is my simple prayer: 'Lord, please help me to have a good biopsy, and I thank you for hearing and answering my prayer.' That is it. Very simple but a powerful declaration of faith, inasmuch as I did not wait to hear the results of the biopsy but immediately upon asking for his help I started thanking Him for answering my prayer. Believing without seeing is what faith is all about. And it works.

If the gift of faith, this driving force behind having a positive attitude, were mine to give, I would give it freely because I know the joy it can put in your heart and the peace it can put in your mind. But all I can do is tell you where to find it. THE REST IS UP TO YOU.

In early 1997, Stranko decided to come out of retirement. He became a part-time consultant for Environmental Engineering Inc. (EEI), a company formed by some of his former co-workers at Ellis and Watts, many of whom he had trained. EEI manufactures the same or similar products as Ellis and Watts. Unlike Ellis and Watts, however, EEI subcontracts some of their work. Stranko works in engineering, manufacturing, and sales. EEI competes with Ellis and Watts.

"I hired the vice president of engineering 35 years ago," says Stranko. "The president had a position in our shop at Ellis and Watts when he first began. I brought him into the office and he moved up to become operations manager. These guys left seven or eight years ago when Ellis and Watts began to downsize."

EEI employs only about 35 to 40 people because they subcontract a lot of the manufacturing processes done at Ellis and Watts. "I was honored to be asked to work here and it makes me proud to work for some of the people I trained," says Stranko with pride. Recently, though, his work was finished at EEI and he went back as a consultant with Ellis and Watts.

Today, he takes care of his ailing wife, Peggy, who is suffering from diabetes and may go blind as a result. He also spends as much time as he can with his family. Stranko volunteers with LifeCenter, helping to promote organ and tissue donation to the public. He still belongs to the Change of Heart support group and often talks to potential heart transplant recipients on the waiting list at University Hospital.

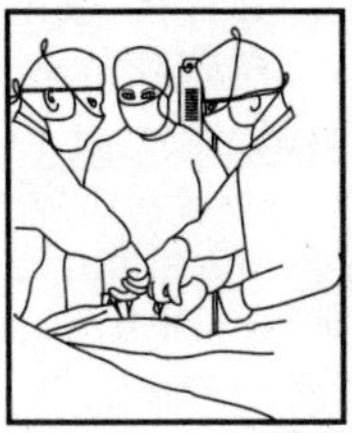

16

Paul Hackman: profile in courage

(Author's note: The following chapter was written in October 1997. Paul died unexpectedly on December 16, 1998. I have written a tribute that appears at the end of the chapter.)

Paul Hackman has faced many challenges over the years. Diabetes robbed him of his sight 25 years ago in 1972 and caused him to lose part of his leg. He says he was granted a new lease on life when he received a kidney transplant on January 18, 1975, at University Hospital in Cincinnati.

Still, in 1996, he watched the Centennial Olympic Games with particular interest and pride. He played a vital role in getting the Olympic torch to its Atlanta destination.

The beauty of the Olympics is that it brings athletes together from all over the world and pushes them to be their best. Hackman has been a longtime volunteer with LifeCenter. He has also been a lifetime resident of Cincinnati. He and his wife, Joyce, now live in Forest Park, a Cincinnati suburb. They have been married for more than 40 years. Joyce is personnel director at Clippard Lab Instruments, Inc., manufacturers of miniature air cylinders and pneumatic valves for control and automation of machines, fixtures, and processes, some like animated figures used by Disney.

Hackman demonstrated true Olympic spirit by overcoming tremendous physical impairments to carry the Olympic torch on June 7, 1996. "It was quite an honor and very exciting," he admits. "The rain stopped just as I began to carry the torch." The torch route was a four-block stretch on Montgomery Road in Pleasant Ridge, another Cincinnati suburb. The runner who accompanied Paul was Brad Zoller, a Wyoming High School student and member of the track team who was to graduate several days later. He had been a student in a health class Hackman spoke to about organ and tissue donation.

"Before Paul's transplant he was near death," says Dr. James Fidler, Paul's transplant surgeon and an associate professor of surgery at the University of Cincinnati College of Medicine. "He had to undergo dialysis treatments five days a week that left him very ill," says Fidler. Twenty-two years later Hackman remains the longest-living cadaveric kidney transplant recipient with diabetes in the world. He is listed in *World Transplant Records*—a publication produced by the University of California at Los Angeles (UCLA)—as the longest surviving cadaveric renal allograft with original disease that may reoccur. In other words, he is the longest surviving kidney transplant patient in the world with diabetes who got his kidney from a cadaver, not from a living donor.

He dedicates much of his time sharing his experience with others, giving talks for LifeCenter to high school students, nursing students, and community groups on the importance of organ and tissue donation. According to Dr. Fidler, Hackman's passion and determination led the Kidney Foundation of Greater Cincinnati and LifeCenter to nominate him to carry the Olympic torch.

Hackman was one of 42 community heroes and nine former Olympians chosen from Greater Cincinnati for the honor. He was featured in several articles in *The Cincinnati Enquirer* and *The Cincinnati Post* prior to carrying the flame.

Before his health problems surfaced, Hackman had been chief accountant at Cincinnati-based Totes, Inc., manufacturer of rainwear gear, boots, and other associated products. By Christmas of 1974, Hackman was on hemodialysis five days a week. From June 1974 until January 1975 his health deteriorated rapidly. "My weight was 105," says Hackman, "down from 140. It was apparent I was not going to live much longer on dialysis. I was sick all the time and sleeping a lot. I couldn't control my diabetes and my blood pressure was very high."

Hackman was in a serious car accident when he was 17. The shock to his pancreas made it stop working. "About a year after the accident I developed diabetes," he recalls. "But from that point on until I was about 32 or 33 years old, I didn't have any trouble with diabetes. Then, everything started going crazy. The diabetes was out of control and my blood pressure was very high."

Hackman saw University Hospital nephrologist Dr. Roy First in February 1974. Talk of a possible kidney transplant was discussed. Dr. First is director of transplant nephrology at University Hospital. "I was at Jewish Hospital under the care of Dr. Ken Kreines, a diabetic specialist," says Hackman. "He thought my problems were related to my kidneys. He wanted to bring Dr. First in to see me."

In February 1974, Dr. First visited Hackman at Jewish Hospital. "He said my kidney function was very, very poor," recalls Hackman. "He said it was about 10 percent of what was normal. I began taking medications for my high blood pressure and water retention, along with potassium, since my level was so low."

By December 1974, Hackman's health was rapidly deteriorating. He was doing poorly on hemodialysis. Dr. First mentioned to Hackman the possibility of a kidney transplant. In the 1970s, diabetics did not do well on hemodialysis. Now they probably do as well as nondiabetics. So Hackman went on the waiting list, even though Dr. First did not give him much of a chance to survive with a kidney transplant.

He received the call that changed his life forever on a bitter cold Friday night, January 17, 1975. His daughter, Vicki, a cheerleader, was at a Roger Bacon High School basketball game. "I had been on dialysis that day and was very sick," remembers Hackman. "I came home and went right to bed. The telephone rang about 11 P.M. It was Dr. First and he said he had a kidney for me. While he was talking to my wife, Joyce, and me, he told us my chances of survival were very slim because of my general health at the time. He gave me (us) one hour to make a decision. It was the hardest decision I've ever had to make. But accepting the kidney was the best decision I ever made. Dr. First said it would be a long operation, about 10 hours. They would remove my spleen and diseased kidneys." The transplant took place on Saturday, January 18, 1975.

After the transplant, Hackman says he felt like he had a whole new lease on life. "I started feeling really good again. My blood pressure was under control. I have not taken any medications for high blood pressure since the transplant. My numbers, creatinine and BUN, which measure kidney function, were really good. The new kidney started working really well. I did go through a mild rejection episode but Dr. First increased the medication and I had a couple of cobalt treatments (standard procedure in the 1970s). The diabetes was under control."

Hackman is especially grateful to the nurses and other physicians who took care of him during his 21-day stay at the hospital. "There were seven of us transplanted that week so there were two transplant patients in one room. The nurses would kid around. It made the days pass very fast. My daughter had a cold and they wouldn't let me go home until her cold was better. When I was first transplanted and in the recovery room, a nurse named Barb who knew I was blind took the time to explain all the medical equipment attached to me."

And his first meal after the transplant? It is something he will never forget. Because his diet was so restricted while on dialysis, his meals and fluid intake were bland and slim. "My fist meal was three eggs, bacon, toast, juice, milk, and all the coffee I wanted. I thought I had died and gone to heaven."

Being on dialysis prior to his transplant meant a strict diet had to be followed—32 ounces of liquid per day, 4 ounces of protein, some fruits and vegetables, but absolutely no salt. "Dr. First wanted to keep my potassium level low," says Hackman.

Being on hemodialysis for more than two months, Hackman had not been able to urinate on his own. The first time his surgeon, Dr. Fidler, had him try, he (Dr. Fidler) had to turn on the water. Coke had a saying, "There's nothing like the real thing," jokes Hackman. "I think they had a kidney transplant recipient in mind when they came up with the slogan."

After three weeks in the hospital, Hackman came home. "I felt good and they took the stitches out the same day I came home," remembers Paul. "I had all kinds of energy. When I first came home I took about an hour nap every afternoon and got some strength back. I started walking around the block in my neighborhood."

Hackman knows little about his donor. "All I know is that he was from Cincinnati. Every morning I say a prayer for the donor and his family. I don't have any idea if the donor family is still alive or still living in Cincinnati. I thank God I'm still alive. And I thank God for the 'gift of life.'"

Through the years, family support has been very important to Hackman. "I wouldn't be here without Joyce and my kids, relatives and friends," admits Hackman. Joyce served as Paul's eyes when he became blind. Hackman attended classes at the Association for the Blind in Cincinnati, learning to get around with a cane and the help of a relative or friend. "I also learned to cook," laughs Hackman. "My family says that's debatable, whether or not I'm a good cook."

Hackman says his kids were really good when he lost his sight. "They were used to playing with toys and leaving the toys on the floor. All of a sudden that had to change. They did very well. I think everyone who is blind goes through some bitterness, saying they'd like to see again. When you go to a football game or a wedding or a baptism, you'd like to see what's going on. I'd certainly like to see my grandkids play soccer or raceball or football, whatever. But my wife is very good at describing to me what's going on the playing field and all around me. When my youngest son, Michael, played football at Roger Bacon High School, Joyce explained each play."

Paul has five children: Vicki, Dan, Steve, Mark, and Mike, and 12 grandchildren.

In 1989, Hackman lost his leg. He developed a disease called Charot's joint. Charot's joint occurs when a joint is damaged by injuries that go unnoticed because of neuropathy, a loss of sensation affecting the joint. Hackman's ankle began to deteriorate, falling down to the bottom of his foot. The whole ankle structure was lost, compounded by severe swelling. Again, diabetes was to blame for this disease. "I went to a surgeon to be fitted for a brace for my leg and it came up to my knee," recalls Hackman. "It covered part of my foot on the bottom and was made of plastic. Unfortunately I got an ulcer on my foot that was treated from September until November 1989. I was in a wheelchair with my foot propped up and Joyce would come home three times a day to clean my foot. I developed an infection on the inside of my foot. The surgeons tried several surgeries to get rid of the infection. For the last surgery, they took skin from the healthy part of my foot and flapped it over the ulcer. That didn't work. I developed gangrene. Dr. Rino Munda, a transplant surgeon at University Hospital, did the first surgery. He cut the leg off right above the ankle." Hackman's foot required a second surgery, this time done by Dr. J. Wesley Alexander, former director of the department of surgery's transplant division at University Hospital and a transplant surgeon. The second surgery turned out well and Hackman's been comfortably wearing a prosthesis since the second surgery.

For the second surgery, after Hackman's foot was amputated, he was in the hospital for about a week. He then received extensive physical rehabilitation for more than three weeks at Holmes Hospital (affiliated with University Hospital). "They taught me how to do exercises with the stump and how to build up my muscles," he says. Then he was an outpatient at Jewish Hospital where he learned things like going up and down steps. "Once that happened, I was fitted for a prosthesis. But there was a long time in between my rehabilitation and getting fitted for the prosthesis." Hackman actually had two prostheses. "One was kind of crude. There was a strap around the waist to hold it up. I started using it and began to walk a little bit. Eventually, I was fitted with one that is below the knee. It works fine now. I have two prostheses. One is for every day use and the other is water repellent. I can take a shower or go swimming in that one."

Hackman still walks with Joyce and other friends and family members around the neighborhood and tries to get other exercises in when his schedule permits.

He was instrumental in helping get legislation passed in Ohio in 1975 that made a provision for individuals to donate organs and tissues when they renew or receive a new driver's license. House Bill 650 needed an impetus to help get it passed. Dr. First told Paul he needed help to make more people aware of this vital community service issue. "I called the local TV stations in Cincinnati and WLWT-TV responded. They came out to University Hospital to interview me. That was the beginning. Eventually, our message was on all three local Cincinnati TV stations." In September 1975, Hackman and Joyce wrote an article for the pictorial section of *The Cincinnati Enquirer*. John Gilligan was Ohio's governor. "The article made its way to Columbus and was attached to House Bill 650 when the governor signed it," recalls Paul proudly. "That put into law organ donor stickers on Ohio driver's licenses."

Shortly after House Bill 650 was signed, Hackman began promoting organ and tissue donation in Greater Cincinnati. For more than 22 years he has been a volunteer with LifeCenter. "I went to about three or four high schools in the fall of 1975," remembers Hackman, "talking to health, science, and religion classes." Today, at age 58 (in 1997), Hackman gives more than 75 presentations to high school, college, medical and nursing students. He also talks to community and civic groups.

In 1978, Hackman was asked to become a member of the Kidney Foundation of Greater Cincinnati. "I've been on the board ever since," he says with enthusiasm.

When Hackman reflects on his longevity with a transplanted kidney, you can see gratitude in his smile and demeanor. He has dedicated his life to promoting organ and tissue donation. Many high school students who hear Hackman speak on the topic make the decision to donate and tell their families. Some have died tragically, becoming donors.

"I never thought I'd live more than 20 years with the transplant," says Hackman honestly. "Especially when the doctors said there wasn't too much of a chance that I'd survive at all. But all of a sudden 23 years have gone by and my kidney function is still very good. In fact, the numbers are about the same as they were 23 years ago when I was transplanted." Hackman still must take insulin daily for his diabetes. "I still feel great. Hopefully I can do the same things I've done in the past."

In the spring of 1998, the Points of Light Foundation named Hackman a Daily Point of Light recipient for May 22. The awards are given daily by the Points of Light Foundation, the Knights of Columbus, and the Corporation for National Service.

When asked about retirement, Hackman says he just wants to keep active. "To not do anything would be such a waste. I want to keep active doing the same things I'm doing now. Joyce probably will not retire for seven or eight more years. I don't know what the future holds. Hopefully my kidney will continue to work. As long as I feel good, I don't see why I can't continue with my volunteer work. It keeps me out of trouble and off the streets." A sly grin and hearty laugh end our conversation.

Tribute to Paul Hackman: remembered as a caring, giving person

Paul Hackman died on December 16, 1998. A devoted husband and father, Paul spoke to hundreds of high school health, science, and religion classes each year for more than 22 years about the critical need for organ and tissue donation, the effects of diabetes and kidney disease, and the prevention of renal failure. As a kidney recipient of 23 years, his story and his courage touched hundreds of students, teachers, and community leaders. His kidney transplant for end-stage renal disease (ESRD) was caused by juvenile diabetes when he was 17. Since his transplant in January 1975, Hackman has been educating teenagers, adults and healthcare professionals about organ and tissue donation.

"Paul was truly a remarkable man who touched the hearts and lives of many people, but none more than mine and his children," says his wife, Joyce, of 41 years. A daughter, Victoria Nesslinger, of Columbus, Ohio; four sons, Daniel of West Chester, Ohio, Steven of Hamilton, Ohio, Mark of Mason, Ohio, and Michael of Harrison, Ohio; a brother, Robert, of Fort

Wright; a sister, Irene Boing, of Jacksonville Beach, Florida; and 13 grandchildren also survive Paul.

The Points of Light Foundation named Paul a Daily Point of Light winner for May 22, 1998. In 1996, he was part of the relay team in Cincinnati that carried the Olympic torch on its way to Atlanta. Also that year he received the JC Penney Golden Rule Award in recognition of outstanding volunteer work.

Much of Paul's time was spent as a volunteer for LifeCenter, the local organ recovery agency for Greater Cincinnati, and the Kidney Foundation of Greater Cincinnati. He gave presentations on organ and tissue donation and renal health in high schools, nursing schools, fraternal organizations, churches, and area businesses, reaching thousands of people each year.

Paul spoke to area high school students about the choice they have to designate themselves as possible organ and tissue donors when they get their driver's license. They were then advised to get their families involved by going home and talking about organ and tissue donation, and the difference it can make.

He also spoke to six-year-old and seven-year-old elementary school children as part of the Everybody Counts program to teach them that people with disabilities should be treated with respect and understanding.

Paul served on the executive board of directors of the Kidney Foundation of Greater Cincinnati for more than 16 years. He also served on the boards of the Clovernook Home for the Blind and Radio Reading Services. Hackman was also a Third Degree Knight with the Glenmary Council of Knights of Columbus #5674.

Even though Paul had juvenile diabetes, was blind, had a kidney transplant, and lost a leg because of diabetes, he continually channeled his time and energy to educate, motivate, and support other members of his community. Even though he was blind, he was a man of great vision. Other people, who are perfectly healthy, claim that they cannot find the time to volunteer. Paul did. And we miss him greatly.

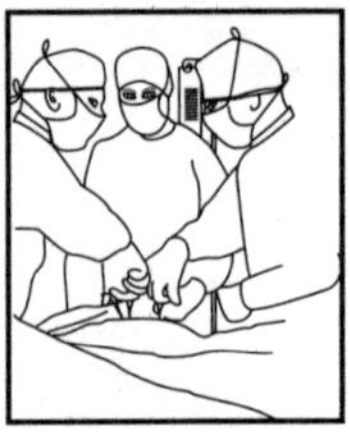

17

Wink White's life is one of determination and miracles

I've known Winston (Wink) White since 1990. Prior to his heart attack and heart transplant, he worked as a truck mechanic for 30 years in Greater Cincinnati. "I worked on forklifts. I worked for Pepsico, Inc., Moon Equipment, and International," he says. White taught mechanics at several local vocational schools and then went to an office job at a uranium processing plant in Fernald, Ohio, close to his home in Okeana, Ohio.

The day White had his massive heart attack he was at home working. He and his wife, Carolyn, a medical secretary in the pulmonary disease department at Good Samaritan Hospital in Cincinnati, have been married more than 36 years. They own five acres of land in Okeana, Ohio, outside Cincinnati. A variety of trees, including fruit trees, dot the landscape, along with a small pond. It is very peaceful. And very quiet.

On November 8, 1988, three days after his 48th birthday, White suffered a near-fatal heart attack. He believes 75 percent of the problem stemmed from his smoking cigarettes. Coronary artery disease also ran in his family. His grandfather died at 48. His father died at 62. On November 8, while working at home picking up rock and two tons of slag (the refuse from metals or ores), White was feeling okay. "I changed clothes a few times and went into the house to rest occasionally," he remembers. "It was Election Day so I went and voted. Then I came home and had the heart attack.

"I took a shower and went to bed and waited until Carolyn came home. She was waiting to vote after work and didn't get home until late that evening, probably after 6:30 P.M. The heart attack happened about 4 P.M."

"Did you know you had a heart attack?" I ask.

"I probably did," says White. "I didn't want to admit it. It was awfully hard."

"Did you have bad chest pains?" I ask.

"One big one. There were pains afterward, but the initial blow was like being hit with a baseball bat. I was numb and had no strength. When I got in the shower I had lost my strength completely. When I went to bed I was still all soaped up. I couldn't even get the soap off me. And I was sweating in the shower. When you sweat in the shower, something is wrong."

White didn't call the paramedics. When Carolyn came home she told him he had to go to the hospital. I said, "I'll just lay here awhile. I'll be all right." Carolyn called a neighbor. The neighbor was rushing White to Good Samaritan Hospital but they decided they had better stop at Providence Hospital (now Mercy Franciscan Hospital-Mount Airy) in Mt. Airy (a Cincinnati suburb), which was closer. "I was at Providence probably 20 minutes before I passed out," says White. "I didn't regain consciousness for three weeks. I'm told I was revived three times with a defibrillator that first night to bring me back." A defibrillator is an electronic device that restores the heart's rhythm. "That night the physicians at Providence gave me about a five percent chance of living if I survived that bout," continues White. "When I woke up three weeks later my chest hurt bad because of the defibrillator. The doctors said they could probably keep me alive for about a year. I told them that didn't sound too good and asked what the alternative was. The cardiologist said he thought I should have a heart transplant." It was still November 1988.

"I asked Carolyn if the cardiologist at Providence was kidding me or what, talking about putting a whole new heart inside me?" recalls White. White asked him what the survival rate would be. The cardiologist told him there was an 80 to 85 percent chance he'd survive the surgery. The national one-year survival rate for heart transplant patients in 1988 was probably slightly less than 80 percent. At University Hospital, the only adult heart transplant program in Cincinnati, the one-year survival rate was in the low to mid 90 percent range.

After a brief conversation with Carolyn, White said, "Well, OK. I guess I just beat the 95 percent chance that I would die, so I guess I gotta' take a chance on the 85 percent chance that I'd survive the heart transplant."

The arrangements were made. The transplant team at University Hospital evaluated White. He was transported to Good Samaritan Hospital in Cincinnati for a cardiac catheterization, one of the necessary tests before being listed for a heart transplant. White was at Good Samaritan for three days. He almost died again undergoing the cardiac catheterization. "I was then transferred to University Hospital where the heart team tried a balloon pump (angioplasty). It was not effective," says White. Dr. David Melvin, director of cardiac transplant at University Hospital, attempted the procedure. White was put on the heart transplant waiting list at University Hospital on December 8, 1988. He was in critical condition, so he was a priority patient for a heart. "They told me they'd probably have a heart for me by Christmas," remembers White. A heart did become available two days after White was listed, but White was too critical to undergo the surgery. He thinks he may also have had pneumonia.

The next day, December 11, White became the first heart patient in Greater Cincinnati to be put on a Novacor®, a left ventricular heart-assist device. White's whole heart was severely damaged. Dr. Melvin, who was in the process of being certified to use the Novacor®, had to call the surgeon general's office to get permission to use the device on White. White recalls Dr. Melvin's words to the surgeon general's office: "If I don't put him on this pump tonight, he may be dead in the morning." So the surgeon general okayed him to do the operation. "He put me on the Novacor® and the following morning the certification came," sighs White. Though he was weary and weak, White was alive. "I hung around on the Novacor® for 72 days," he says, smiling slightly. But the journey to getting a new heart was far from over for White.

White says he knew, for the most part, what was happening around him after being put on the Novacor® by Dr. Melvin, but he did sleep a lot. "I knew I was tied to the bed," says White. Restrained for his own safety would be a better term. The Novacor® did the work of the left ventricle of White's heart. It was inserted into his abdominal cavity and controlled by a computer at the foot of his hospital bed. That was the reason White was tied to the bed. "I was trying to leave all the time," jokes White. "They had to tie me down! Every time I had a chance I wanted to get out of there (hospital)."

On January 16, 1989, another heart became available for White. "I had kidney failure," he recalls. Again, he was too critical to receive the transplant.

White didn't know Dr. Melvin too well at this time. "I didn't know what he was doing," says White. "I thought he was always going on vacations." Today, White and Dr. Melvin are the best of friends. "It seemed like he was never around, but would periodically pop up from time to time. It was probably just me. I was probably just popping up periodically. I had a lot of dreams and was pretty well sedated in the cardiac intensive care unit (CICU)."

Did you think you were going to die? I ask White.

"I wasn't too sure," he replies. "I was going to do all I could to keep from dying, I'll put it that way. I thought I was going to check out a couple of times but they (doctors, nurses, etc.) brought me back."

The Novacor® was saving White's life. But it was uncomfortable. He couldn't sit up in bed. He had to eat lying down. "I wouldn't eat, let's put it that way. Nothing tasted good." White had a catheter in for over four months. He also had to use the bedpan for bowel movements. "I was locked up. You don't eat. You don't go. And I was tied to the bed. The computer was operating the Novacor® that pumped blood through my body. I had tubes and lines sticking out of me everywhere and I couldn't get up."

Being awake on and off, dreaming and other psychological factors associated with long-term illnesses began to take their toll on White. He was fed intravenously. White was intubated on and off for four and a half months. "I was awake sometime every day," he says, "because they'd come in and ask me if I knew where I was." And I'd say, "Yeah, I know I'm in the hospital."

"What hospital?" they'd ask.

"And I'd tell them, University."

"Do you know what time it is?" they'd ask.

I replied, "I don't care what time it is. It makes no difference. I'm here. They covered the clock on the wall anyway. That made me mad all the time. I didn't know what time it was."

The clock was covered because it was where the curtain went. They pulled the curtain and it covered the clock in White's little cubicle. "I didn't really know if it was daylight or nighttime."

White thought the nurses and residents didn't want to take care of him because he was a lot of trouble. "I needed somebody to look after me nearly all the time," he recalls kind of sorrowfully. "I had tremendous bedsores and my legs were stiff. They had to put casts on my legs to keep my feet bent so they wouldn't lie down (drop foot). I had to wear the casts about 18 hours a day. I had a hole being rubbed in the side of my leg from the tube that came from the computer wires being taped there and I kept ripping that loose. It was a huge hole in my right leg at the knee. They kept taping it back and I kept ripping it out. Today I have a scar that's about 1 inch wide and 2 inches long from the hole that the wire put there."

Somehow in the transfer from Providence Hospital to University Hospital White lost his false teeth. "We never did find where they went," he says smiling. "I didn't get teeth until I was discharged in May 1989."

On February 7, 1989, another heart became available for White. Again, he was too critical to receive it. "Everybody was hoping I would get a new heart for Valentine's Day," remembers White. "Wouldn't that have been appropriate? It didn't happen."

After 72 days on the Novacor®, White finally received a new heart on February 22. It was Washington's Birthday. "I had received my 'gift of life,'" says White thankfully. "I thank God, my donor, and his family for this second chance at life."

White's recovery was slow, though the heart was an excellent one. "I had little strength because my body had deteriorated so rapidly," recalls White. "I had no voice because of the long intubation in the cardiac intensive care unit (CICU). Every time they'd take the respirator out, it seemed

I couldn't breathe and they'd stick it back in. They'd tell me to just open up and then I'd swallow that tube down and I was done."

"The anesthesiologist said he was no problem," recalls Carolyn. "He would just say open your mouth and his vocal chords would just go (gestures apart)."

But White wasn't allowed to have a drink of water. He could not have eaten anything even if he had wanted to at this time. He was still being fed intravenously. Before the heart attack, White weighed 150 pounds. After the transplant he weighed 116 pounds.

White's long hospital stay did have a few amusing moments. He says when he was in the CICU the nurses would never give him a call button. "When I had one I used to buzz it all the time," he remembers. "So they took it away from me. I'd sit there in my room and I didn't have any teeth and I'd try to whistle with my little fingers in my mouth (motions with fingers). I could hear the nurses sitting and talking at their station and they'd say, 'He's whistling again.' One would say to the other, 'Well, he's your friend, you go see what he wants.' Then a nurse named Carol Dunn would come in. She always took care of me."

Carolyn interjects, "The nurses loved him, Jeff."

"I hated Lynn," replies White with a coy smile. (When I had my heart transplant I had Lynn too. She was the weekend nurse in the CICU.) "She took my lunch, didn't she? She took my sandwich."

"He was somewhere else," says Carolyn. While he was in the CICU, he had ICU psychosis for four and a half months. He had many strange dreams; he also had these dreams when he moved to the step-down unit.

But Lynn actually saved White's life about four times in the CICU, "with resuscitation and stuff," as White puts it. "I'd tell my wife, 'I don't want to be here this weekend. She's going to be here. And she does not come in here when I need her.' And she was always there when I needed her, you know. I dreamt about camping with one of the nurses and we were in the rain. And I gave her hell one day when she came in my room, for letting me camp in the rain."

White also had dreams about Dr. Melvin. "He would make these little statues out of us heart recipients and he'd wind them up and they'd walk, run, you know. And he'd get the biggest kick out of that. I had this one dream about him transplanting a black guy. It must have been Luther (Luther Watson, who was transplanted shortly after me in 1989)."

"Luther was after you," interjects Carolyn.

"And this black guy got this heart and he got in his room and he jumped out the window and ran around the hospital and then came back," recalls White vividly. I said, 'Damn, if he can do that, I can do that! So I would jump out the window but I couldn't make it around the hospital.' I don't know how that dream ever ended up."

One day White called a nurse in to his room and said, "I'm getting out of bed!"

She said, "Where are you going?"

White said, "I'm checking out. I'm tired of being here. I'm leaving."

And the nurse said, "You can't leave!"

"And they'd use harsh language with me."

Carolyn interjects, "Oh, yeah, right!"

Ceil said, "You try to get out of that bed and I'm going to smack you down."

I said, "You ain't smacking nobody. I'd tell them to get Carolyn on the phone, and I'd tell her, 'Carolyn, my damn car is sitting down in front of the hospital running. Somebody's going to steal it. Nobody knows how to drive a stick shift. I got to get it moved.' Then I'd call the nurse and say, 'Do you know how to drive a stick shift car? I need my car parked. It's down in front of the hospital running. I was getting ready to check out and you wouldn't let me leave so'... I had a lot of goofy dreams like that, but the cutest one was the one with Dr. Melvin winding up these toys."

White says that one day Ceil came in to his room and he had a dream where he was swimming under water and collecting seashells and selling them.

"You used to tell me they took you to therapy at four in the morning and made you go swimming," says Carolyn to Wink.

"Yeah," he replies.

"At four in the morning," asks Carolyn incredulously.

The nurses said, "Where are you going?"

White said, "I have to go to rehab. They want me to go swimming."

"You ain't going anywhere," they said.

"One time I was going to check out of the hospital."

"Where are you going now?" the nurses asked.

I said, "Well, my mother died and I have to go to her funeral! I don't think anybody ever told my mother that."

One day Carolyn came into White's room to visit. "I gave her hell," he says. I said to her, 'Where have you been? Here I am sitting on this seashore and I got all these shells to sell and I've only got one hand. I ain't got enough hands to do what I gotta' do!'

"No," interjects Carolyn. "You had two hands but you needed three!"

I said, "Where have you been? I needed you here. Now I'm stuck with all these seashells and everybody's calling me! Where I came up with these dreams I don't know. But the dreams probably played a part in keeping me alive."

White says when he was moved to the step-down unit he not only had 24-hour nursing care but he also had a sitter around the clock. "If I went to the bathroom," White says, "I couldn't come back out without somebody helping me. The nurses and the sitter were real good. They would rub my feet and massage my legs and stuff like that. I guess they were like my sisters after awhile. To this day they are still amazed that my transplant worked out as well as it did. The nurses told Carolyn about three times that I was going to die, and that if I were living in the morning it would be a miracle. They were never supposed to tell Carolyn anything. Dr. Melvin had given them strict orders not to communicate any information whatsoever to her. But he made himself pretty available. I mean, when Carolyn called him, he was there."

White had one male nurse named Mike Krueger in CICU. "He was pretty good," admits White. "I was always asking him for a drink of water. I used to have this dream in the CICU that he and I were fighting a war and we were fighting to stay alive, you know. And I'd say, 'Can I have a drink of water?'"

"No, you can't have any water today. Your bucket's got a hole in it and it won't hold any water so I can't give any to you."

"I'd ask him every day, 'Will you patch my bucket so I can have a drink of water?'"

"Maybe tomorrow. Maybe tomorrow."

White remembers the day he was extubated (the respirator was removed). "While they were taking the tube out, I thought there was a big ocean liner passing outside the hospital window," recalls White. "The doctor was pulling that tube and I'm thinking, man that boat is moving slow! It's taking forever for this tube to come out. When the tube came out, the boat passed on by. That's what was going through my mind. It just seemed like it took forever to get the tube out. I don't know how long it takes."

After White's heart transplant he received weekly biopsies. "Yeah," says White. "Down in the cath lab they all played the piano and sat around and sang and talked, whatever. Those are the things I thought. I'd lie on the table and they wouldn't do nothing. They'd all gather around in little coffee klatches, talking, and I'd say to myself, gosh dang, I'd wish they'd start and get it over with. I couldn't lay that long because my rear end hurt so bad from a bedsore."

Shortly after the transplant White developed an infection and they couldn't find the cause of it. "They did a computerized tomography (CT) scan of my whole body and found a guide wire had been left in me from a previous biopsy."

They had to get that wire out of White. "The next thing I know," says White, "I was on my way down to radiology or the cath lab. They made an incision and I was awake for this deal. I'm lying there and being attended to by a female doctor and a little foreign doctor, two of them. The female doctor tries to grab this wire, OK, and they cut this little slit. She's poking around down in there saying, 'I can't reach it. I can't reach it.' Make the slit bigger to get down there because I'm really hurting laying here. Finally she got hold of it and said, 'I got it! I got it!' And this little foreign doctor said, 'You got it? Pull the goddamn thing out of there!' That's exactly what he said. And she pulled it. It broke. Then they had to dig around some more. Finally they got it out and wheeled me back to my room. It was just one of those things."

"It's just one of those things," says Carolyn mockingly. "They were going to pull all of his teeth because they couldn't find the cause of the infection." White had false teeth that were lost en route from Providence Hospital (now Mercy Franciscan Hospital-Mt. Airy) to University Hospital.

"They were going to pull the teeth I had left," says White. "Then Carolyn called my dentist and he talked them out of it."

"They were going to pull them all," says Carolyn. I said, "No, that's it."

The guide wire caused the infection. It wasn't until September or October, after he'd been home since mid-May, that he got a new pair of false teeth. At that time, he did have an infection in his gum from one of his back teeth. The cyclosporine, an immunosuppressive medication, caused White's gums to grow over the teeth left in his mouth. "An orthodontist had to cut my gums away," recalls White. "I literally walked around with band aides on my gums for three or four days. After my teeth healed, I went and got fitted for new false teeth. They were nice."

In the CICU, White says he had "this big black transporter whose name was Lorenzo. He was good too. If it hadn't been for him, I wouldn't have been able to get up at all. I mean he'd come into my room and just pick me up and get me standing while holding onto me. I'm not supposed to tell you this story. I'm not supposed to tell anybody about this. These two nurses, both of whom were named Becky, got me out of bed one day and then I was taken to physical therapy. Physical therapy brought me back to my room but the only people around were Becky and Becky. They couldn't lift me to get me in bed. I was in a waterbed because of bedsores. So they said, 'Well, we'll throw him in bed.' And they both just grabbed me, counted to three and threw me in bed!"

"No they didn't," Carolyn interjects. "They got you over on the nightstand and Becky, who was pregnant, hit you with her belly."

"Well, whatever," replies White. "I went in. They (the two Beckys) said not to tell anybody they did that and I couldn't wait to tell Carolyn what they did to me. But being in intensive care wasn't real bad. I had to have the sheets changed a lot. Did you ever have a sheet changed while you were laying in bed?" he asks me.

"No," I reply. "I never did."

"That's a hell of a job," says White. "They roll you over one way and pull the sheet out and then roll you over the other way and pull the sheet out. It's even rougher when they put the new one on the bed. I had four and a half months of that stuff. I always had a wet bed. They'd take the catheter out and tried a few other things but I still ended up peeing in the bed. When the catheter was finally taken out for good, I was so used to having it in that when I had to pee I'd just go in the bed."

Carolyn offers another amusing anecdote about the time Dr. Melvin, Joe Reising (a cardiothoracic surgeon at University Hospital then), and Mike Krueger got White out of bed because he wanted to stand up and go home.

"I told Dr. Melvin," recalls White, "that I want out of here. I can't stand this. Get me up, God . . . I can walk and stand and do . . ."

Dr. Melvin said, "You don't have enough strength to stand up!"

White said, "Well, I bettcha' I do. So he and Dr. Reising had Mike bring in my cowboy boots because they had high heels. All three of them had a hold of me and they put my cowboy boots on and I'm standing there with their help."

Carolyn says, "You should have seen him. He only had on his hospital gown and cowboy boots! His catheter was still in him."

According to White, Dr. Melvin said, "Do you think you can stand up here now?"

White said, "You're damn right. You just turn me loose and watch me!"

So they said, "OK, are you ready?"

I said, "I was ready. And they turned me loose and I just peeled down to the floor like a wet noodle, man."

Dr. Melvin said, "I told you you wouldn't be able to stand."

"Put me back in bed," I said. "Damn. I couldn't wait to get to bed. And then I accused Dr. Reising of leaving my boots in the rain. He and I got along pretty good though."

Dr. Melvin had White's wires (for defibrillation) pulled out shortly before he went to the step-down unit. "I thought, Oh, Christ!" says White. "They're going to cut on me some more. But it was simple. They just had a resident come in, grab the wires, and jerk them out."

White stayed in the CICU until the second week in April 1989 before he went to the cardiac step-down unit. "I was in CICU for a month after my transplant," he says. "When they were getting ready to take me out of CICU they had to use a slant board to bring me up gradually because I had been laying in bed so long. They'd get almost completely vertical and I felt like a limp rag. I'd beg them to just lay me back down. They'd come back every day with the slant board and tip me a little further until I was straight up. It was to get me used to standing again. Your muscles atrophy after laying in bed so long with no exercise."

When he went to the step-down unit in mid-April, White had to begin physical and occupational therapy. Actually, he went to physical therapy several times before going to the step-down unit. "I had to go to physical therapy for rehabilitation. It hurt. I didn't want to do it. I'd do anything at all to get out of it. I was so weak. I had no strength. I couldn't stand up. I couldn't walk. It took me three weeks to walk with a walker. The therapists then let me walk with a walker for three days, took the walker away, and gave me two canes. Then they took one cane away and let me walk with only one cane."

"Who was down in physical therapy with you who told you to quit feeling sorry for yourself?" interjects Carolyn.

"Ed Luebbe," says White. "He's the one that really got me to walk. I started to use the parallel bars." Luebbe was the ninth heart transplant recipient at University Hospital. He has since died. But he had had two hip replacements after his heart transplant. "They were trying to get me to walk the length of the parallel bars, holding on to each one. I was standing there one day and this guy (Luebbe) was sitting in his wheelchair. I didn't know him but he knew me. He looked at me and said, 'You can do that, Wink! Come on! I know you can do that!' And I just picked up my hands and walked across that thing and man, I made it to the end. It was only six feet, not very long. I just grabbed the bars. I found out Luebbe was another heart transplant recipient and was down there getting rehabilitation because he got a hip replacement. After that I started walking around the hall."

"Then they'd take you to occupational therapy and make you wind a rope up with a 2-pound weight. It felt like it weighed 50 pounds. I could hardly push a 2-pound weight up a board. I had a whole in my stomach after the Novacor® was removed. They couldn't close it so they left the hole to heal on its own. In the beginning, they packed a whole roll of gauze inside it. Gradually it healed. I could tell it was healing because they'd peel a little off the roll and stick it in each time. The roll kept getting smaller and smaller."

Physical therapy was long and hard for White. "Sometimes it hurt so bad I could have cried," he admits. "I hated it. But I went one day because they wouldn't let me use the toilet. I had to go on the bedpan." I said, "Damn it, I want to go on the toilet." They wouldn't let me. When I went down to therapy they let me use the toilet, but then I couldn't come out of the bathroom. I was stuck there! And the people in therapy would have to go get somebody to get me out. Still, White persevered in spite of himself. "With the help of an excellent therapist, my mother, my wonderful wife, and a strong will to succeed, I completed the task."

Says Carolyn: "What about the girl from occupational health who used to come in your room and ask you to add. She'd come in and ask you what two + two was."

"Yeah, it was seven," jokes White. "Hell, I didn't care what it was. I flunked the math test."

He said, "I ain't stupid. I just can't walk," remembers Carolyn.

"They asked me all these goofy-assed questions you know, to see if there was any brain damage," says White. "I guess I flunked pretty bad. I must have had a lot of brain damage but it turned out pretty well because I still know that 2 + 2 is 4. But if you go any higher than that I'm out of luck," he says facetiously.

For most of his hospitalization, White had little or no appetite. Even when he went to the step-down unit none of the food looked or tasted good to him. He was even put on the hospital's five-star menu which offered food like breaded shrimp and chicken cordon bleu. "I had this black gal for a sitter," recalls White. "She looked hungry. I'd say to her, 'Would you like this? It looks pretty good. Why don't you just take it to the waiting room and eat it?' And she'd take it up there. Then the dietician would come and say she wanted me to drink Ensure®, a dietary supplement. I was supposed to drink four or five cans a day. I had a refrigerator in my room full of Ensure®. The dietician would ask how I liked it and I'd say it's good. I love it."

"What flavor do you like?" she'd ask.

White said, "Chocolate and strawberry. I didn't want no vanilla. And that black gal would come in and I'd tell her to bring a bag and go to the refrigerator. See all that stuff (Ensure®) in there? Put it in your bag and carry it out today. Take it home and let your kids drink it. I never had an appetite for eating anything. Carolyn even brought me Skyline (Cincinnati) chili and coney islands, my favorite… But nothing tasted good."

White says it wasn't until his last two weeks in the hospital that he really started to eat. "It was sometime toward the end of April," he says. When he was in the CICU he continued to lose weight. He says he was told he was burning 2,500 calories a day just lying in bed. "They couldn't pump enough juice into me to maintain any kind of body weight. My legs were the size of my arms. I asked Mike Krueger a couple of times in CICU if he thought I was going to walk again. He smiled and said, 'Yeah. You probably will.' He was pretty inspirational and made me believe I would get better. For awhile there, I wasn't sure if I was going to get better or not, to be honest."

White had quite a bedsore on his tailbone. The nurses kept it packed and tried to let it heal. By the middle of May 1989, Dr. Melvin decided to let White go home. The media was also interested in White's discharge. "Dr. Melvin asked if I would do two interviews on TV and radio. I was real fine that day until I got up out of bed and had something, like bone or calcium stuff break loose in my inner ear and I became real dizzy. I got sick and could only lie on one side. But I managed to get through the interviews and Dr. Melvin asked if I could walk out of the hospital. He wanted me to walk out the front door. I said I'd try. After the interview I got up and focused on the front door. I held my two canes up, went for the door, and then put them down. Everybody was gathered around, hanging out the hospital's windows up in CICU. Carolyn came with the car, picked me up, and I went home. I really didn't heal until September, so it's a good thing they didn't keep me. I'd probably have gone crazy. I already thought I had found a second home the way it was."

About a month after he came home, his employer, Fernald, also interviewed White. "They wanted a picture of me with my truck (White has a 1951 Ford pick-up, a show truck). I wanted to be Joe Cool and put my leg on the bumper of the truck for the picture. Well, it only took three people: one to hold me up and two to put my leg on the bumper for the picture. They got the picture for the employee newsletter."

White never did return to his desk job at Fernald. He has been on disability since his transplant and took an early retirement.

About a month after he came home from the hospital, White finally got his new teeth. Life was not all that easy, though. "I sat around the house while Carolyn was at work all day," he recalls. "My mother came and stayed with me a week."

The night I interviewed Wink and Carolyn was March 29, 1997, Easter weekend. How does White feel about his experience, his second chance? "Here I am eight years later still pulling some punches," he says with a grin. It was a long and painful ordeal for him. "I don't have a word for the whole experience. I think I went through a bigger ordeal with my health than most people. In six months I probably had more pain and suffering than a lot of people have in a lifetime. But I'm here. I mean, I'm alive. That makes it a good experience." He celebrated his 10-year transplant anniversary with a "White Christmas in July" on July 24, 1999.

White's seven-month hospital stay and heart transplant cost almost $1 million. His daily immunosuppressive medications cost about $1,400 per month while his other follow-up care like regular lab work and quarterly heart biopsies cost approximately $26,000 per year.

In 1991, two years after his heart transplant, Carolyn made arrangements for White to meet his donor's family after corresponding with them. They live in Hillsboro, Ohio. The donor, a 24-year-old named Rodney Holiday, was killed in an automobile accident, a head-on collision. He had multiple head injuries and was transferred to University Hospital. "I think Carolyn and the young man's parents were both in the surgical waiting area at the same time," recalls White, "but they didn't know each other. And then Dr. Melvin came out and told Carolyn they had a heart for me. He said he just had to go to the operating room next door to recover it."

Today, Wink and Carolyn still see the young man's family. White has a photograph of him. The family owns a grain and feed store in Hillsboro. Rodney had taken over the business when he was killed. "You look at her (his mom) and you know she would rather be talking to her son," says White with a hint of sorrow. "And that's what I told her. I can thoroughly understand."

Rodney was a very good photographer according to White. "He liked to photograph animals, especially dogs," says White. "He was a pretty witty kid."

Then White recalls something rather strange. "One day in the CICU, after the transplant, Carolyn came into the room and while I was half sleeping I looked at her and said, 'Call me Rodney.' She said, 'What did you

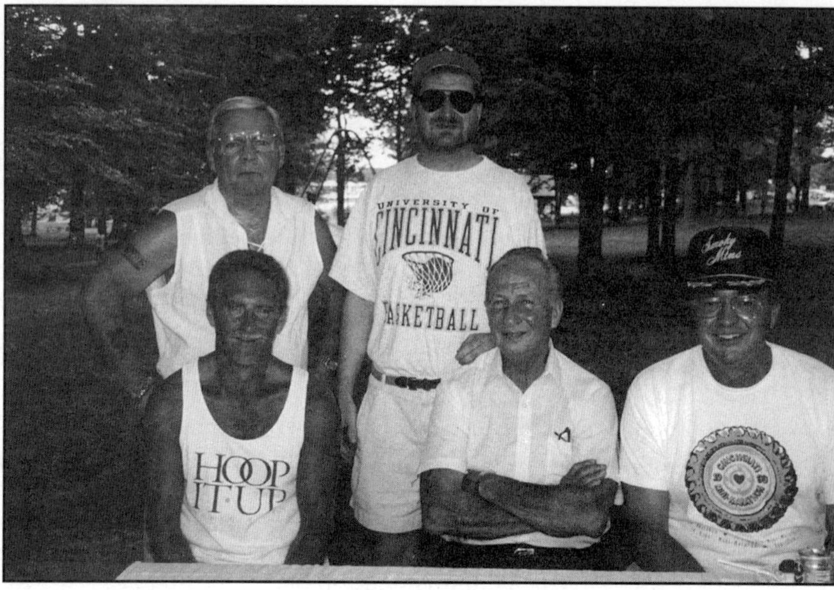

Celebrating 10 Years

Heart transplant friends of Jeff Lueders at his 10th heart transplant anniversary picnic. *Seated from left to right:* Greg Osterman, Jack Stranko, and Ken Robertson. *Standing from left to right:* Wink White and Jeff Lueders.

Photograph © by Debbie Lueders

say?' I said, 'Call me Rodney.' That was really strange. How that name came to me I don't know. I didn't even know I really said it until Carolyn told me. Then I found out the donor's name was Rodney!"

The only rejection White had with his new heart was the first day he was home. "They wanted me back in the hospital," he says. "Well, you can tell them they ain't getting me! I ain't going back. I was there long enough." A hospital nurse came to his house several times to give him intravenous injections of prednisone.

White has only been in the hospital one time since his transplant. "I wasn't feeling well and Carolyn took me to Mercy Franciscan Hospital-Mt. Airy. I woke up and there was this nurse that I didn't really recognize but she was one of the nurses during my first nights there after the heart attack. I told her I had to get out of there because I had tickets for the Jimmy Buffet concert and I couldn't miss that. So I got out of the hospital that next morning and went to the Buffet concert that night.

"I've been very lucky. Somebody upstairs is on my side. Plus a lot of people down here. I had a good cardiologist. A good surgeon. It all adds up to life I guess because I'm still here."

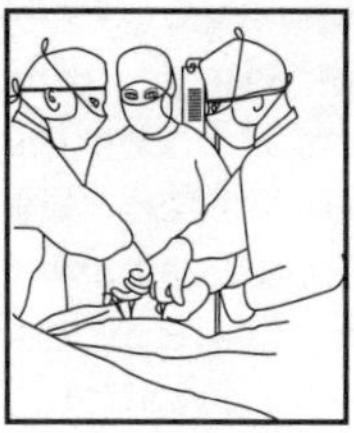

18

Transplantation and donation are family affairs for Craig and Connie Steele

For Craig and Connie Steele of Reading, a Greater Cincinnati suburb, the 1990s have been filled with medical miracles and tragedy. Still, the family has fought through the tough times. Now, they are enjoying the good times.

Their daughter, Ashley underwent two liver transplants at Children's Hospital Medical Center. Her first transplant was January 15, 1992. Seven months later, on August 31, she received her second liver transplant from a five-year-old child from Florida. She suffered from biliary atresia, a disease affecting the liver's bile ducts. Though she suffered from vanishing bile ducts, she was very active for two years after her second transplant. She was walking and talking and playing with her older brothers, Terry and Nathaniel. Connie says, "She was a dainty eater and she was smart as a whip." On May 28, 1994, Ashley died of pneumonia and other complications related to her liver transplant.

But the Steele's story does not end here. After Ashley's transplants, Craig, then 35 and a facility maintenance employee at Johnson & Johnson's Ethicon Endo-Surgery in Blue Ash, a Cincinnati suburb, was on medical leave and on peritoneal dialysis at home, waiting for a kidney/pancreas transplant at University Hospital. He went on the waiting list in October 1993.

Craig had been a diabetic since he was seven. In the year leading up to his being listed for a kidney/pancreas transplant, his blood sugar levels were very high. "I was losing energy and just not feeling well," he relates. He was first put on hemodialysis but "it left me physically weak and depressed. I felt like I was losing my mental dexterity. I was close to suicide," he admits.

For the next five months Steele was on peritoneal dialysis and did very well. On February 26, 1994, Steele received a kidney/pancreas transplant. The organs he received were from Elizabeth Sherlock of Loveland, Ohio, who died of an aneurysm. "I was free from being diabetic after the transplant," says Steele, who no longer has to take daily insulin shots. "I felt human again. I had a better quality of life. The transplant was a second chance for me." Steele met James Sherlock, Elizabeth's husband, at a tree-planting ceremony in Winton Woods Park in Cincinnati in April 1994.

In 1995, Steele lost his transplanted kidney. But on February 23, 1995, in a living unrelated transplant, he received a kidney from his wife, Connie. Although somewhat rare at the time, donation by a spouse is becoming more common. Steele has returned to his job at Ethicon Endo-Surgery. The Steeles' sons, Terry and Nathaniel, are now grown. And the Steeles have a new toddler, three-year-old Cameron. Craig and Connie Steele are ardent volunteers with LifeCenter, helping promote organ and tissue donation.

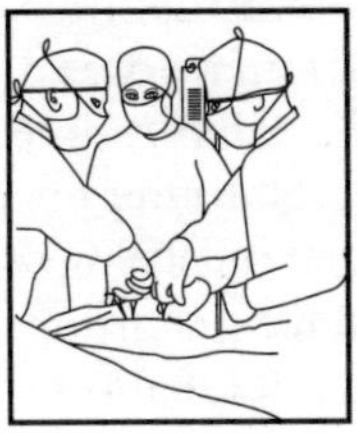

19

Ed Lowe: a physician becomes a patient

When Dr. Ed Lowe came into this world on March 1, 1938, it was nip and tuck for about a year. "I was a premature infant weighing a little over three pounds," says the pediatric physician. "But I came through fine."

Dr. Lowe was born at Cook County Hospital in Chicago, Illinois. His family moved to Cobert, Michigan, a small town in southwestern Michigan, when he was four. It was there, on a small farm, that Dr. Lowe grew up.

"My father was born in Mississippi and raised in Arkansas," says Dr. Lowe. William Edward Lowe came to Chicago in his 20s and met his wife, Mildred (Millie). She had been born in Arkansas but raised in Chicago.

During World War II, William was in the Signal Corps. He developed a love and vocation for radios. In high school, he studied the plumbing trade. From there, he attended Arkansas A&M College in Pineville. When the war ended, Dr. Lowe's father worked on the assembly lines of the automobile plants in southwestern Michigan. But he developed a serious lung condition working in these plants and had to get out of that environment to save his life. So he started his own plumbing business and radio repair shop. He continued in the plumbing and radio business until his retirement. "When I was in high school, college, and medical school that's what my father did," says Dr. Lowe proudly. The first time he retired was in 1969. A year and a half later he became the plumbing inspector of Inkster, a Detroit suburb of 55,000 people. Dr. Lowe is equally proud of the fact that his father was the first African American to become a member of the state plumbing board and the inspector's board for the state of Michigan. He was also the second African American in Michigan to get his master plumber's license.

Dr. Lowe and his family—he has a sister, Elaine Elizabeth Jenkins, two years younger, who is a licensed practical nurse (LPN) and a nanny; and a brother, six years younger, Matthew Alexander, who has a construction business in Los Angeles—grew up on a farm. "It was a small farm," relates Dr. Lowe. "We raised our own fruits, vegetables, and animals for our own consumption. We did sell fruit on the side."

Dr. Lowe went to Cobert High School in the Michigan town where he grew up. He graduated in 1955. From there he went to the University of Michigan. His freshman basketball coach in high school convinced him to go into a scientific field, because at the time there weren't that many opportunities for minorities in business. "I originally wanted to be a dentist," he confesses. "But I decided in my second year at Michigan to go to medical school instead. He graduated from the University of Michigan in 1959 with a degree in zoology. He then entered medical school, graduating in 1963. I was going to become a pediatrician, but because of the Vietnam War, I ended up going into anesthesiology, and ultimately into pediatric anesthesiology. The latter was deferred to finish my specialty training. Then I went into the service and served in the Philippines during the Vietnam War."

From 1967–1969, Dr. Lowe served at Clark Air Force Base in the Philippines. The hospital was a 350-bed in-patient hospital and two thousand bed-holding unit. There were 74,000 people on the base. The base was the first stop for the wounded in the Medevac chain. Wounded soldiers in Vietnam were Medevaced to mobile army surgical hospitals (MASH units), then usually to medical ships then to the Philippines.

"I didn't think we should have been in the Vietnam War," says Dr. Lowe candidly. "But that was not for me to question. My job was to take care of patients and that's what I did. I saw a lot of trauma and a lot of tragedy, but I did come out with a feeling that the human body is a very resilient thing. The reason it was so resilient in the patients I saw was because they were young. I was there to do my job."

When Dr. Lowe returned to the States in 1969, he joined the staff of the University of Michigan's Department of Anesthesiology as associate director of pediatric anesthesia at Mott Children's Hospital. He stayed for two years, coming to Children's Hospital Medical Center (CHMC) in Cincinnati in 1971.

Dr. Lowe's wife of more than 40 years, Alice, is a retired nurse. They met when Dr. Lowe was in medical school and she was a med-surgical nurse at the Veterans Administration Hospital in Dearborn, Michigan. "I met Alice through my sister and her brother," says Dr. Lowe. "We were married when I started my internship."

The Lowes have two children, both of whom live in Cincinnati. Son Cedric is a chemical engineer with A.M. Kinney and is actively involved in Young Life, a Christian organization dedicated to young people. Their daughter, Shannon Rousch, and her husband own an architectural firm.

Dr. Lowe says the reason he chose Cincinnati's Children's Hospital was because he was looking for a job that was less administrative and more clinical. "It was also close to my parents in Michigan," he says.

Dr. Lowe's first experience with transplant surgery occurred in 1965 at the University of Michigan. He was involved in several early adult heart transplant surgeries at Ann Arbor when he returned from the service in 1969. "When I came to Cincinnati I was involved with both donors and recipients as an anesthesiologist for renal transplantation. I've been involved in both since that time."

Dr. Lowe's role of talking to families about donation began when he became more involved in the intensive care unit (ICU) in 1984 at Children's Hospital. "I broached the subject, discussing the aspects of organ and tissue donation with families. I was very involved with that as co-director of the ICU, calling LifeCenter transplant coordinators in as early as possible."

In the April 1993 issue of *Health Care Review*, a former Cincinnati health newspaper, Dr. Lowe is quoted in an article written about him as saying, "It's difficult for physicians to broach the subject of donation when you work closely with a family. You are affected by the closeness that develops and that affects your ability to ask. You're asking at a time when the family is in grief. It's tough. However, one must work through that. I've always found it productive to take my resident with me to ask for organ donations. It teaches them how to do it. There's a certain way of approaching the family. It's something that must be taught.

"Most of us as human beings are very caring individuals and when it comes to being close to people who are experiencing a tragedy we find it difficult to impose upon them at a time when that tragedy is occurring. In order to do this, it is not a gift but something that is learned. The only way residents are going to learn to do it is to be exposed to it and be in the presence of someone who has learned to do it. If possible, it's not something you want to do by trial and error."

That was in 1993. Today, clergy and LifeCenter transplant coordinators request organ and tissue at CHMC.

Working in the ICU and operating room at Children's, Dr. Lowe saw all his patients that came through the ICU after an organ transplant. "After having seen many of them when they were very sick, it was very gratifying to see these children getting better. But many of them went through difficult times before they felt better. To see a child who had liver disease so bad that you didn't know if they were going to die this moment or the next, get through the perioperative period and walk out of the hospital, was very gratifying."

Dr. Lowe also worked on organ donors. He saw grieving families though he knew he was helping someone else. "Again," he reiterates, "it is a learned response. I learned the response many, many years ago as a junior medical student. My first experience with death left a lasting impression, and actually left me with the question of whether I was going to continue in medicine. I had a long talk with a close relative who said to me, 'You will face this the rest of your professional life. You learn to live with it now or you need to get out of the profession.' I learned it then and to impress upon you how much I learned it, when I sat at the funeral of my grandfather, with whom I was very close, I felt no emotion at all. I knew I had probably overlearned what I'm talking about. That has sustained me, even to this day, in those situations. It didn't really scare me because it was a learned behavior. That doesn't mean I couldn't feel for the family."

Dr. Lowe was diagnosed with cardiomyopathy in September 1990. He noticed several of the symptoms while skiing that spring in Colorado. "I thought I was in pretty good shape even though I wasn't getting any regular exercise. I didn't have the time. I was working 16 to 20 hours a day." For a year and a half, he was treated with medication—digoxin, captopril, and lasix—by cardiologist Dr. John Schneider. Dr. Lowe's ejection fraction improved from about 17 percent to 28 percent.

Dr. Lowe says he felt pretty good until he went to Michigan for a few weeks following his mother's death the week before Memorial Day in 1992. He worked until the first of May. "I went to her funeral and took care of her affairs," he remembers. "Then I found it difficult to absorb any food or walk any distance. When we came home, I couldn't walk across the room."

University Hospital's cardiac transplant program determined he needed a new heart. He checked into the hospital for a cardiac catheterization on a Thursday and was put on the waiting list for a new heart the following Tuesday. In the hospital, he developed severe congestive heart failure. He was in the CICU when he was awarded an Excellence in Teaching Award two days before the transplant. Ten days after it was determined Dr. Lowe needed a new heart, he received one from a 22-year-old from Hamilton, Ohio. The doctor had become a patient.

"Having dealt with transplant patients as an anesthesiologist, I knew where I was," says Dr. Lowe. "I knew I had one chance of surviving, of living. I knew it even more the day they took me to the hospital when I couldn't even walk across the room. I knew if I didn't have a heart transplant I was going to die."

So what kind of patient was he? "My philosophy is simple," he says. "I find that I have always wanted to be the type of patient that I wanted my patients to be. I know I know a lot, but I also find that it's a lot easier on the people who take care of me if I act just like any kind of patient. I find that difficult to do sometimes but I keep it to myself. For example, for a nurse to come in and tell me, 'Dr. Lowe, you need to take your medications, or Dr. Lowe, you need to put pressure on the site of the cath if you should start bleeding, or Dr. Lowe you shouldn't lift so and so.' I find that it grinds me sometimes, but I keep it to myself. I have a tendency to be the type person who keeps things to themselves. And I have a very long fuse. I do not consider myself a difficult patient. If I have a concern, I will voice that concern in a way that I hope is not at all degrading or comes across questioning the thought process or ability of my caregivers, be they doctors, nurses, lab techs, or any one. That is my philosophy."

Dr. Lowe had two serious rejection episodes in the first year of his transplant. The episodes were serious enough to require a burst of steroids the first time and IV steroids the second time in the hospital.

Dying did cross Dr. Lowe's mind. "When I started to go downhill in March 1992, I would have periods of depression, wondering if I was going to die. But once I got the transplant, that seemed to go away. Since the transplant, my greatest concern has actually been, believe it or not, how long will I live and should I continue working the way I work now or should I just hang it up and start doing some of the things I enjoy. I remain ambivalent about that."

Since his transplant, Dr. Lowe has resumed his normal workload. He was forced to give up his clinical work because of the risk of infection and now works as a professor of clinical anesthesia and pediatrics at the University of Cincinnati College of Medicine. He also directs the residency program in anesthesia at the College of Medicine and is on the admissions committee. Dr. Lowe now devotes about 80 percent of his time at Children's Hospital to administrative work, while 20 percent is spent teaching.

Dr. Lowe enjoys teaching, which he has been doing since 1967, for several reasons. "I enjoy exploring and learning myself," he admits. "I get a great deal of joy out of giving material to trainees and then witness their progress. My philosophy of teaching is everyone should be brought to his or her potential. That potential may not be the same for everyone, but whatever that potential is, my job as a teacher is to develop it." Dr. Lowe teaches both medical students and residents. "No student should be embarrassed in front of the class."

Still, like every heart transplant recipient, Dr. Lowe worries too. "I do think on and off, depending on just how tired I am or what I'm doing, about rejection and infection. I fear both."

Before Dr. Lowe was diagnosed with cardiomyopathy in 1990, he had several patients at Children's Hospital in the ICU who had Coxsackie virus, a virus that attacks the myocardium causing a viral myocarditis or pericarditis. This may be how he contracted cardiomyopathy. Cytomegalovirus (CMV), which can cause enlargement of cells of organs, often affects those with transplanted organs. It can be deadly. Dr. Lowe is CMV negative, meaning he is at great risk for CMV. "It's very surprising that I'm CMV negative because I've worked exclusively with children since 1969," he says with dismay.

Dr. Lowe says he is very grateful to the donor and donor family. "I often wonder who it was," he admits. "I was given the opportunity to have my life extended."

A member of the advisory board of LifeCenter and a fervent volunteer in helping to promote organ and tissue donation, Dr. Lowe often works behind the scenes. "I'm a very private individual," he maintains.

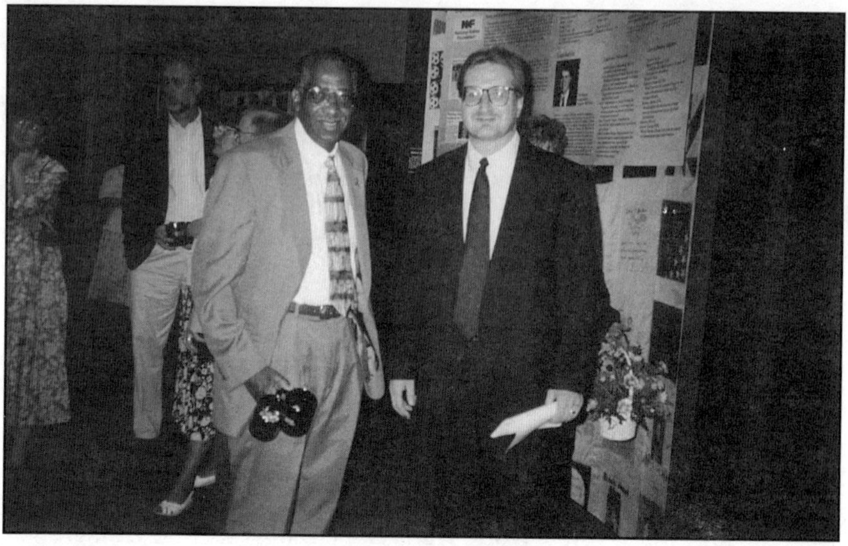

Celebration of Transplantation

Fellow heart transplant recipient Dr. Ed Lowe and Jeff Lueders at Celebration of Transplantation, June 9, 1998, at Cincinnati's Museum Center.

Photograph © by Debbie Lueders

Certainly he is an inspiration to his students. Residents tell him he works as hard as anyone when he could be sitting around enjoying life. "They like to hear my story," he says. "They like my dedication and drive."

Dr. Lowe is very personable. There are no small people in his eyes. "Every person from the most important to the least supportive is important to me. Until you show me otherwise, I will always look upon the positive aspect of your life."

Through it all, Dr. Lowe's wife, Alice, has stood by him. She was very happy about the transplant but it was also stressful for her. Uncertainty can be daunting. Alice keeps up her nursing license with continuing education units (CEUs) by volunteering at nursing and retirement homes like Maple Knoll. She is on the board at Twin Towers, one of Cincinnati's largest retirement and nursing communities.

Dr. Lowe continues to work 10 hours or more a day. He exercises daily on the treadmill and walks in his Springfield Township neighborhood near Winton Woods, a Hamilton County park. "I've recently decided not to take work home on the weekend." He smiles and graciously shows me to the door.

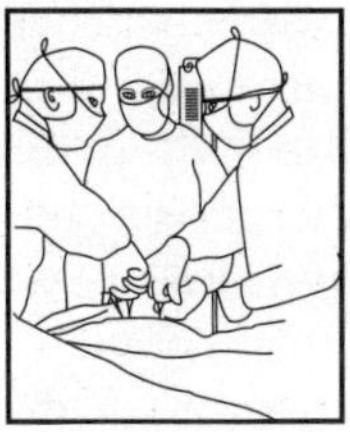

20

Georgine Wolohan: community volunteer and so much more

Georgine Wolohan had never met anyone who had had a liver transplant. But on a hot, humid day, July 23, 1986, she was about to receive one. In Pittsburgh, Pennsylvania. As a former nurse educator who had worked at the Cleveland Clinic and at Cincinnati's Good Samaritan Hospital, Wolohan knew about organ transplants. "It (a liver transplant) wasn't something that caused me to open my arms and say 'whoopie,'" she recalls.

Wolohan's onset of liver disease began slowly in 1969, when her son was about a year old. She had hepatitis. It seemed to come and go, she says. "I guess I thought it was gone but occasionally I'd turn yellow and be very tired. I'd go to the doctor, he'd run blood tests and there would be the elevation of the bilirubin." Bilirubin is a reddish yellow pigment occurring in bile, blood, urine, and gallstones which is useful in determining the nature of certain liver diseases. "That's where it seemed to stay," she continues. "In 1976, I was sent to the Mayo Clinic and put on a drug called penicillamine. The diagnosis was primary biliary cirrhosis. I was monitored every four months but I had a good life. That went on for about 10 years. I lived with the knowledge that there was no cure for my liver disease. By 1986 I was in the final stages of liver failure. My bones had become so brittle they were cracking from merely rolling over in bed. In June 1986, getting ready for my son's high school graduation, I was running down the stairs of our house when I tripped and broke my hip."

Wolohan was treated for about a week at Bethesda Oak Hospital in Cincinnati. "That's when I knew a liver transplant was the only thing left to do." She would have to go to Pittsburgh.

On June 23, 1986, the day before her birthday, Wolohan was taken by ambulance to Cincinnati's Lunken Airport to a medijet bound for Presbyterian University Hospital in Pittsburgh. Dr. Thomas Starzl, a pioneer in the field of liver transplantation at Pittsburgh and before that, at the University of Colorado in Denver, evaluated Wolohan. The rest of her organs were still in good shape. She was put on the United Network for Organ

Sharing (UNOS) list. Her coping skills proved she could handle an uphill fight. Her wait began. She was a candidate for a liver transplant. She also had hip replacement surgery at Presbyterian University Hospital.

"While waiting in the hospital, my husband, Tim, stayed with me. He and my children never let me believe I was not going to make it. I watched their eyes for signs. Friends from the Junior League in Cincinnati called and sent notes of encouragement. One, Chris Stubbins, then the organization's president, brought me a mascot. It was a teddy bear. Friends drove up and back in a day to see me. Bear was dressed in a fashionable Junior League T-shirt, pearls and white gloves. Bear and I had conversations during long lonely nights. I received more love and support than any one person could fathom."

Since Tim is a self-employed commodities trader, he was able to stay with Wolohan the entire three months she was in Pittsburgh.

As a nurse, Wolohan felt she was much more aware of everything going on around her at Presbyterian Hospital. "Nobody was going to do anything to me unless I fully understood it," she says matter-of-factly. "But the staff was very good about explaining everything to me. I was lying in the hospital waiting for a liver transplant while recovering from hip surgery. I was out in the hall every day and down in therapy trying to learn how to walk so that when I got the liver I'd be able to make it. I had pain from my hip, but I didn't have a lot of pain from my liver problem. It was just a lot of itching, jaundice, swelling, not bad physical pain. It was not an easy first month in the hospital."

At 1:00 P.M. on July 23, 1986, Wolohan got the call that would save her life. It came through on her hospital telephone in her room. There was a donor match. "The voice on the other end of the telephone said, 'There's a liver for you,'" recalls Wolohan. "I was so excited. I had my crutches by my bedside because I could hardly walk. I started to cry. I went out to the nurse's station, and after a month I knew the staff real well. I said, 'I've got a liver!' I mean, it was my chance for life, to make it. Without that I was going to die. I had real mixed emotions. I remember vividly the nurse coming in and the anesthesiologist saying, 'Well, we're going to prepare you now, but in the event this is not a good match…They're getting it now in Tennessee and if it doesn't turn out you know, you won't necessarily get it.' There was the realization that someone else's heartbeat had stopped. I was just a heartbeat away."

A woman down the hall from Wolohan who had had primary biliary cirrhosis also came to Wolohan's bedside to talk and offer support. She'd already had a liver transplant. "I kept thinking, well, she was older than I am and look, she's made it. I really did just put my hands in the Lord and I just felt that I was going to make it."

Dr. Starzl and his team gave Wolohan all the confidence she needed. "He'd come in with his entourage, different doctors and the transplant coordinator from the hospital, even the orthopedic doctor that performed my hip replacement. They kept saying things were going great, you're going to do it." Wolohan was number eight hundred and something at Pittsburgh to receive a liver transplant. She doesn't know what number she was.

But she does have strong feelings for the parents of a teenage girl from Tennessee—her donor family. Their daughter died in an automobile accident. "I will never understand the loss, the feeling of abandonment, the grief they experienced while making their decision to donate," says Wolohan emotionally. "I say a prayer of thanksgiving for them each day. I know they are comforted in the knowledge that good has come from their tragedy. I do not know their names but they are my heroes.

"No potential organ recipient wishes ill upon anyone, but tragedies do occur, that is a certainty of life. I believe organ donation is a profoundly spiritual act—the highest act of charity in recognizing that all human beings need one another and have an obligation to help one another."

Wolohan was 45 when she had the transplant. The toxins in her system made it difficult for her to use "the basic tools of my personality—words. 'Lots of words,' my husband Tim always said. My eyes and skin were so jaundiced, I appeared more green than yellow."

During September 1986, Wolohan stayed in Pittsburgh so she could get follow-up care at Presbyterian Hospital. She was on a myriad of immunosuppressive medications to combat the rejection of her new liver. For the first seven years after her transplant, she returned each year to Pittsburgh for an annual checkup. She has not gone back to Pittsburgh for the last seven years.

By the beginning of October 1986, Wolohan was finally able to go home. She had to recover not only from the transplant and a bad case of rejection, but also from her hip replacement. She suffered from steroid psychosis. She was so pumped up with steroids to combat the rejection that she lost touch with reality. "It was a little struggle getting back, until they lowered the dosage," Wolohan admits. "But I've still got the same liver, thank God."

In April 1987, Wolohan went to Vienna with Tim to visit her daughter, Tara, who was studying abroad. She began to resume her normal lifestyle almost immediately. She worried about being around people with colds or the flu, because she didn't know what would happen. To organ transplant recipients, a cold can be deadly if not treated properly. "In the beginning," says Wolohan, "I did worry a lot about getting a cold or the flu. I went home with a booklet that said if you have vomiting or any of a list of symptoms, you should take extra precautions."

In the mid 1980s, Wolohan was one of the founders of the Organ and Tissue Donor Awareness Council of Greater Cincinnati. The council sponsored month-long activities in April to promote organ and tissue donation in Greater Cincinnati. She was chairman of the council in 1988, obtaining permission from Nabisco, Inc., to use their LifeSavers® logo in campaign materials. Her picture was also on a brochure promoting organ and tissue donation that was used in the Ohio Bureau of Motor Vehicles (BMV) for those who renewed or received a new driver's license and wished to become donors. The council disbanded in 1996.

Also in 1988, for Cincinnati's bicentennial, Wolohan was named one of two hundred Great Living Cincinnatians.

Today, 14 years after her transplant, Wolohan is healthy, works as a freelance writer, and as a docent at the Cincinnati Art Museum. She is also a former Woman of the Year in Cincinnati and is involved with many community activities, including helping to promote organ and tissue donation with LifeCenter. "I just take the opportunity to make sure people know where I've been and where I'm coming from, and that life is certainly worth living," says Wolohan hearteningly. "I'll always be on immunosuppressive medication daily and am more susceptible to infections than the average individual."

Every July 23, when Wolohan gets feeling that, "Wow! God, this is my transplant anniversary!" she knows a family in Tennessee is not having the same kind of day. "Their memories," says Wolohan prayerfully, "are of someone (a daughter) they loved who is gone. I hope they say to themselves she is living on in others."

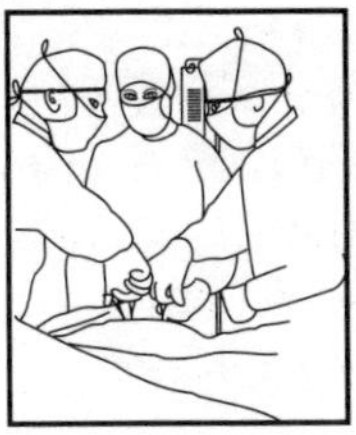

21

Building memories through faith and family

For liver transplant recipient Dale Merz, every day is Father's Day. "I live my life for my wife, Mary Kay, and my kids," says the 44-year-old Green Township resident. "Anytime I can spend more time with my kids makes me happy." And it makes them very happy too. Dale and Mary Kay have seven children: Adrienne, 19, who's in college; Renee, 17; Stacie, 15; twins Dale and Diana, 13; and twins Brian and Lisa, eight. School, camping, soccer, and baseball keep the family busy. Dale is a carpenter with Bambeck and Vest, a construction company that specializes in office remodeling. Mary Kay, who received an education degree from the College of Mount Saint Joseph, teaches sixth grade at a local elementary school.

Dale's health problems began when he was about 19 years old and developed ulcerative colitis, which severely damaged his colon. At age 25, he required an ileostomy, a surgical formation of an artificial anus by connecting the ileum to an opening in the abdominal wall. About this time, Dale also developed sclerosing cholangitis, which caused the bile ducts in his liver to clog and collapse. The disease is a rare condition in which all the bile ducts inside and outside the liver become narrowed. His liver was severely damaged. No treatment was available other than a liver transplant.

"By July 1988, Dale looked and felt worn out, tired, and had lost a lot of weight," says Mary Kay. "He always gave 100 percent but until the transplant it just wasn't enough." Dale received his liver transplant on August 1, 1988. Dr. Israel Penn, Dr. Jean Tchervenkov (a transplant fellow at the time) and Dr. Mark Epstein, a resident who rotated on the transplant service at University Hospital, led the surgical team. "When Dale went through his transplant experience, I knew he was desperately sick," continues Mary Kay.

By July, when Dale was so ill, Mary Kay had to rush him to the hospital where a battery of tests were done, including an endoscopic retrograde cholangio-pancretography (ERCP), a procedure in which dye is injected into the liver's bile ducts to test function. "The doctors couldn't even get the dye in," recalls Mary Kay. "It was supposed to be an outpatient test. But Dale was very disoriented and did not know who he was or what he was doing. He was running a high fever and was becoming more and more yellow. We knew transplant was in the picture, we just didn't know when. I never thought about the transplant until the team of doctors came in to talk with us. At that point, it was too much for me. I turned it all over to God. I couldn't have imagined what I would have done without God, having five little ones." Dale and his family attend Our Lady of Lourdes in Westwood. Though they were all very young, Dale and Mary Kay's five children did visit him in the hospital.

"I thought it would be a fairly routine operation and I'd be home in four to six weeks," says Dale. "I knew I needed a transplant and I had to have it to get better. When I was in the hospital, I never even thought about the cost. And dying never crossed my mind." Health insurance covered the transplant, follow-up care, and immunosuppressive medications. His old liver was the size of his fist according to Mary Kay. "The doctors couldn't understand how he was getting around with such a damaged liver."

Dale's recovery was long and arduous. He was in the hospital for three months. "I think I had every side effect there was: pneumonia, lymphoma, hematoma, and cytomegalovirus. When I came home, I had cataracts, a hernia, and chicken pox. I was off work for about a year. While I think I taught my doctors a lot, I really appreciate what the doctors, nurses, and other staff did for me."

Dale came home on October 22, 1988. The day after Thanksgiving he was back in University Hospital with chicken pox. "All five little ones then came down with chicken pox," says Mary Kay. "Between Thanksgiving and Christmas, we had five kids with chicken pox. Dale couldn't come home until the last one was over them. We brought him home on Stacie's birthday, December 23.

"We tried to be a family again. I remember us sitting in the living room that Christmas (1988). The kids were opening a few little presents. They didn't seem to notice they didn't receive huge presents that year. Dale and I just sat there thinking it doesn't matter. This Christmas is the best. It didn't matter what presents were under the tree, just that Dale was here in this house with all his kids. No present we could have given him was better than that."

The last 12 years have been very good to Dale. "I can't complain a bit." He has lab work every two months at University Hospital and continues to take his immunosuppressive medications daily. "I have good stamina. I could work more than 40 hours a week but it would take time away from my kids. When I was young, I used to think 44 was old. Now that I'm 44, I don't feel that way at all." Eight years ago, Dale and Mary Kay had their second set of twins, Brian and Lisa, now eight.

Since Dale treats every day like Father's Day, this June 18 (2000) will be no different. He will be spending it with his family. "I try to succeed as best I can to show my appreciation to my donor and donor family. I believe that's the reason, in the long run, that God gave me the transplant. So I can take care of my family."

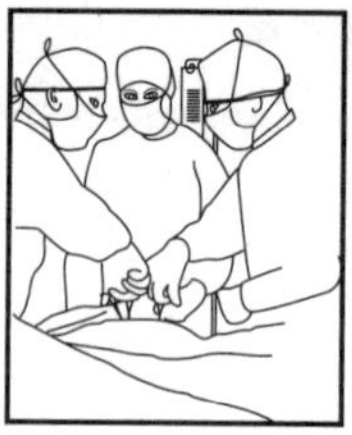

22

Strong family and positive attitude helped former burn patient survive

Though it happened 26 years ago when he was eight, Mark Rogers vividly remembers the spring day he was burned severely over 83 percent of his body—his torso, arms, legs, face, and hands. The burns were third degree.

Today, at 34, Rogers has been happily married for 14 years, has a rewarding career, and a three-year-old son, Stephen, and a one-year-old daughter, Renee, both of whom he adores.

The road from near-death had many, many curves—endless surgeries, pain, and stress. Through it all, Rogers never lost faith in God and was surrounded by a loving family and medical staff at Shriners Burns Hospital who never gave up. More importantly, Rogers himself never gave up.

Rogers remembers the day it happened like it was yesterday. It was April 17, 1974. The weather was fairly warm. "We all had on long pants and short-sleeve shirts." He was in the third grade at St. Vincent De Paul School in Riverside, a Cincinnati suburb.

"I went up behind our house into the woods where my brother, Mike, then 15, was up there with a neighbor," recalls Rogers. "They had a can of gasoline and had found an ax head with wood chips still in it. I saw what they were doing and started to leave. Someone threw a match; it went out. Then someone threw one that went in the gasoline can our neighbor was holding. The neighbor threw the can. I happened to be going down the hill when he threw it. It hit me. I was badly burned.

"I started to run and my brother and neighbor tackled me. I was just so hot. They tried to roll me. I ran down to my house. The first thing you're taught when you're young is to go to Mom when you're in trouble. When I got in the house, I couldn't stay still from the pain. I took off outside. That's when my brother and neighbor picked me up and threw me over the fence into another neighbor's swimming pool.

"We were waiting for the ambulance and I asked my mom if I was going to die and she said, 'No!' I asked her several times and she said, 'You're going to be fine.'"

"After that, I never did question my injuries, though I heard the doctors talk about how bad I was. I just knew all along that I was going to make it."

Rogers was rushed to General Hospital, now University Hospital in Cincinnati. Dr. Edward Law, who was assistant chief of staff at Cincinnati's Shriners Hospital, saw Rogers at General Hospital and did not expect him to make it. But he told Rogers' parents, Ed and Martha, if he made it through the night and stabilized the next day, they would move him to Shriners.

The next day he was transferred to Shriners. This began a four-month hospital stay. "First of all," says Rogers, "I was given no pain medication. I learned to accept the pain, even though it was excruciating. But my parents and older brothers—Mike, 15, Dave, 14, and Al, 11—kept a positive attitude. The doctors and nurses at Shriners were always positive too. They never showed any signs of giving up. Everybody was like family. They all helped me a lot mentally."

"When I first saw Mark, I didn't know what to think," says his mother, Martha. "I had never seen burns like that. When Dr. Law talked to my husband, Ed, and me, he told us right out, 'He's a big burn. I can't guarantee anything.' You had to take things one day at a time."

Shriners Hospital in Cincinnati is owned and operated by the Shriners Hospitals for Crippled Children (SHCC). It is a national network of 22 hospitals—19 orthopedic units and three burn institutes. All offer specialized medical care to children up to age 18 with a full-time staff of 360. Many, like Rogers, are followed up to age 21 for reconstructive surgery. Shriners Hospital opened in 1922 and since then more than five hundred thousand children have received specialized care in Shriners' hospitals through the philanthropy of this fraternal organization. No payment is ever sought or received for treatment from the family, the U.S. Government, or any third-party payer for services rendered in Shriners Hospitals. The hospital system is supported by the SHCC Endowment Fund, which is maintained by contributions and bequests from Shriners and the public.

Shriners specializes in acute and rehabilitative care of burned children. The 30-bed Cincinnati unit serves children who live within a one thousand-mile radius of Greater Cincinnati. An average of 225 acute admissions are handled yearly, 50–75 of those locally or regionally.

The Cincinnati unit now has 14 acute/intensive care beds and 16 reconstructive/rehabilitation beds. Acute patients are those with newly acquired burn injuries. Reconstructive/rehabilitation patients are those needing surgery or therapy to increase their functional ability and physical appearance. Dr. Glenn D. Warden, chief of staff, who joined Shriners in 1985, now leads patient care.

Rogers endured countless skin grafts with donated skin from Ohio Valley Tissue and Skin Center (OVTSC) in Cincinnati. He thanks God every day for the donors whose skin saved his life. The cadaver allograft skin was used to cover the burns and protect the body's deeper tissues from injury, drying, and invasion of foreign organisms. Cadaver skin helped regulate Rogers' body temperature, fought infection, helped with metabolism, alleviated pain, provided excretory and absorbing powers, and contained peripheral sensory nerve endings. Skin has limited regeneration abilities. No regeneration occurs with third-degree burns. Small areas of Rogers' skin healed with granulated tissue covered by a thin epithelium (cellular tissue). Rogers' life could have been threatened by serious fluid loss and rampant infection had his open wounds not been covered, cleaned, and closed by donated cadaver skin. Dr. Law and Dr. Bruce McMillan, who later became chief of staff at Shriners, treated Rogers. Both burn surgeons performed his skin grafts and reconstructive surgeries. Physically, Rogers was in bed for three months before ever getting on his feet. "Three days a week I was in the operating room."

Edward C. Robb, chief operating officer of OVTSC and the Intermountain Tissue Center in Salt Lake City, was working as a Shriners researcher when Rogers was a patient there in 1974. Since infections presented a serious problem in severely burned patients like Rogers, Dr. McMillan, and Robb and Paul Nathan of Shriners developed a synthetic barrier dressing to cover Rogers' burns. It was a spray-on system that effectively isolated the thermally damaged tissue from microbial contaminants derived from Rogers or the environment.

At Shriners, the LD-50 has risen greatly over the years. LD-50 refers to the percent burn at which 50 percent of the patients die. In 1971, three years before Rogers' accident, the LD-50 was 39 percent, meaning that if the total body burns of a patient reached 39 percent (of the body), half of them would die. Today, the LD-50 is 85 percent, meaning that if the total body burns of the patient reach 85 percent, only half of them will die. In 1974, Rogers beat the odds through determination, faith, and a positive attitude, greatly reinforced by his excellent medical care at Shriners. As Dr. Warden likes to emphasize, "Every child who doesn't die at Shriners is a success story."

For the first year after Rogers' accident, Dr. Law and Dr. McMillan operated on Rogers completing almost 50 skin grafts, using his own healthy, unburned skin on the burned areas. This protected the tissue beneath the skin and helped the new skin look more normal.

While in Shriners, Rogers remembers the twice-a-day baths in the whirlpool. "They reached right under my back and I had no skin there," he recalls. "They'd put you in the whirlpool and scrubbed you raw. If they had donated skin to put on you they did a dressing change and bandaged it up. If it was a spot that was going to be left open and not have skin on it, they would just put ointment on and bandage it up. It was sheer hell! I had one nurse, Betty Waters. We called her Grannie. Her saying was, 'Mark, you don't have to want to go, but you're going.' After I got better, it was a joke, but it's the truth. Every night I knew when my mom and dad left what was coming. And I'd tell them, 'Don't leave.' There are things in life you don't want to do but you have to do them. Grannie invited my mom and dad to stay one night and watch. Mom didn't want to watch but dad stayed. He was holding my wrist and the blood was just running down my hand." Rogers endured this twice-a-day treatment for four months until he was released.

Rogers is sure his parents and family knew the odds of his survival. Rogers believes he was one of the fifth or seventh largest burn patients ever to live at that point. "I lucked out because I had no internal injuries. I didn't swallow any fumes or flames or smoke so my lungs were fine," says Rogers. "It was just the outside."

Rogers admits Dr. Law was brutally honest with him and his family regarding his chances of survival. While he and the nursing staff remained optimistic, Rogers' burns were quite severe. "Dr. Law's famous words were, 'He's a big burn. He's here today, but we don't know about tomorrow,'" says Rogers. "He was straight forward. Once a week the doctors had meetings where all the parents of burned kids could attend. He went around one by one and addressed your child and how he or she was doing. Every week my parents would come back and I'd say, 'What did he (Dr. Law) say?' The meetings took about a half hour away from visiting hours. They'd come back and say, 'Well, it's the same thing you know. You're a big burn. You're here. You're progressing, but you're not out of the woods yet.'"

During Rogers' four-month hospitalization in Shriners ICU, his parents could visit him, but his brothers could only come on Sunday and look at him through the glass since he was in isolation. Rogers' parents had to be masked and gowned to go in his room. "My brothers would always come up with something stupid like making faces through the window. But they made me laugh and let me know they were there. Sometimes I couldn't even see them. I called home every night. If the neighbors knew I was on the phone, they'd come running over to our house to talk to me."

Rogers admits the burns he suffered drastically changed his looks. But it wasn't a severe psychological blow. "I never did worry about what I looked like after the accident," remembers Rogers. "From day one my parents, my physicians, and nurses at Shriners told me, 'All that counts is what's inside!' If people can't accept you, if they don't look at you on the inside first and only look on the outside, then they're not your friends. I never did worry about it. I got out of the hospital on August 29, 1974. The first place I went was McDonald's. Two weeks later I had to return and stayed until October 1. The moment I got out of the hospital the second time, I wanted to go right back to school.

"I learned I was no different than anyone else and had to face the fact I almost lost my life. My appearance changed. I don't try to hide it. A year after I was out of the hospital I started to play organized baseball again. I learned if I wanted to do something, I just had to set my mind to it."

Rogers returned yearly to Shriners until 1986 for cosmetic surgery to improve the appearance of his scars. "I went to clinic at Shriners at least once a week," recalls Rogers. "Each time in clinic there would be 40 or 50 kids so you got to see someone that you hadn't seen in a couple of years. At least once every year I went in for reconstructive surgery."

Rogers' first surgery released his chin from his collarbone because his chin had grown over to his collarbone. Other surgeries included both legs, arms, neck, fingers, and underneath his knees. "I was really fortunate my hands didn't get burned a lot," says Rogers. "Neither did my feet."

Living in Cincinnati with a Shriners Hospital saved Rogers life. "Had I lived somewhere else I probably wouldn't have made it. And anytime they had a cancellation for reconstructive surgery, they'd call me to see if I could come in. I could get in Shriners, have the procedure, and get home a lot quicker."

Over the years, Rogers made friends with many other patients at Shriners. He was the first president of the Burn Support Group and stayed involved with the group for about four years. "Every time I went into the hospital I'd meet different people. Invariably, every time you left you had someone you wrote to all the time. When I was first admitted in 1974, I met a girl who had no brothers and I had no sisters. We adopted each other. Until 13 years ago when her father passed away, her family lived in Kentucky. She and her mom moved to Florida and I haven't heard from her.

"Every year when you went into the hospital you always tried to get in at the same time as someone you knew because you had so much fun with them. It was a friendship with someone in the same situation as you. You knew from year to year what they went through. Many times I went to Shriners to talk to parents and kids to encourage them. Nurses would ask me to read to the kids in the ICU."

In May 1997, Rogers and his family attended the 75th anniversary of the Shriners Hospitals. In 1994, he and his family attended the 25th anniversary of the Cincinnati burn unit. "That was really neat because they brought in a lot of patients and nurses I knew," he says. "There were probably 30 patients and doctors and nurses I hadn't seen since 1979. You lived with these people for long periods of time. They were family."

During his four-month hospitalization at Shriners, Rogers kept up with his studies with a tutor. "A nurse or my parents would flip the pages for my reading assignments. I missed nothing as far as school was concerned."

Besides studying, TV took Rogers' mind off the intense pain. "Having the nurses and doctors and my parents in the room with me also helped," says Rogers. "I didn't sleep a whole lot because they'd wake you up constantly. I was fed high protein milk shakes. Every half hour they gave me a 16-ounce milk shake."

As for eating, to keep his metabolism regulated, Rogers had to eat as much as he could. "Dr. Law once told my dad I had to eat the equivalent of what a lumberjack eats," he remembers. "I never was a big eater but at Shriners I'd eat four helpings of everything. They would shove peas on a fork and feed them to me when I was on my stomach. I'd eat anything they put on my plate."

By early October 1974, when he was released from Shriners after a second one-month stay, Rogers returned to school at St. Vincent De Paul in Riverside. There were 70–80 kids in the school. "We all grew up pretty much in the same neighborhood so I fit right in," recalls Rogers. "No one ever teased me or made fun of me. If anything, the other kids helped me."

When he got to Elder High School, a lot of kids had questions and asked what happened. They were positive questions. How did the accident happen? What were the circumstances?

Though Rogers had to wear leg braces, he still managed to play organized baseball. He was asked to play for Elder but declined. He had a chance for a baseball scholarship at Kent State, but decided he wanted to be employed full time.

"I was only allowed to take my braces off when I was active, like playing baseball, swimming, or other sports," says Rogers. "Otherwise, I had them on 24 hours a day. I loved sports, so that was one way to get out of wearing the braces. And it kept me in good shape. Now that I look back, the leg braces weren't so bad. You're restricted but wearing braces was something I had to do or I wouldn't get better."

Faith played a large role in Rogers' recovery. "A priest from General Hospital and one of the priests from St. Vincent De Paul gave Rogers communion every Sunday when he was hospitalized. Their encouragement always included keeping the faith. "I was always brought up to pray every night before going to bed," reflects Rogers. I still do. As I get older, my prayers seem to get longer. There's no doubt in my mind that the guy up above knew I had to be left here for a reason. I beat the odds of surviving with such severe burns. So there had to be somebody pulling for me."

Rogers graduated from Elder High School in 1983. He went to work for Kohl Packing Inc., meat packaging plant. He started as a grunt and worked himself up. Within a year, he was supervisor in the packaging room. He worked there for seven or eight years until the company was sold to Kluener Packing Co. Rogers delivered furniture for a year. Then he got a call from Ed Kohl, the former owner of Kohl Packing. He went back to work for Kohl at Kluener as a sanitation supervisor and then a shift production manager. "They wanted me to move with the plant up north from Cincinnati, but I told them it wasn't feasible." Rogers was married in November 1986, and his wife, Denise, works at Factual Data near downtown

Cincinnati. Today, Rogers is packaging supervisor at Queen City Sausage. He has been there eight years.

"Denise was from our neighborhood," says Rogers about his wife. "I had known her all my life. She hung around with my cousins. We thought we really didn't have much in common. Her dad actually coached me in baseball for a couple of years. Before you know it we were dating in April 1985 and then got married."

In April 1988, Rogers' mother, Martha, was put in the hospital for congestive heart failure. In January 1989, she was transferred from Mercy Franciscan Hospital-Western Hills to University Hospital in Cincinnati. Dr. David Melvin, then director of cardiac transplant at University Hospital, told her a heart transplant was the only thing that would save her. She stayed in University Hospital until the end of April, receiving her new heart on April 1, 1989. Martha was the 72nd heart transplant and I was #73. We became great friends.

In talking about his mother, Rogers maintains that sometimes the patient is better off than the family in a serious health crisis. "Not because of the pain and suffering, but sometimes it's easier on the patient than it is on the family," says Rogers. "In my case, both mom and I were the ones laying in bed and we're not totally altering our schedule to get to the hospital. Mom and I are as tight as any mother and son can be, because we ran to Shriners all the time and every day she was there for me. Her heart problems were hard on the whole family but I think I worried and prayed more because of how close we were. When we look back, my situation probably helped us because we had been through so much and knew how to cope with health problems. We knew the best thing for mom was family support. For her entire hospitalization, there was not a day that I did not get to the hospital to see her. I knew it was that important. I knew she was close to death."

Five years ago, Martha Rogers suffered another setback. She had breast cancer that required a mastectomy. She had the surgery and again the great support of her family. She has been fine since the mastectomy.

Dr. Richard J. Kagan, director of the burn unit at University Hospital, assistant chief of staff at Shriners and medical director of OVTSC, says that success with a patient such as Mark Rogers is not defined while the patient is in the hospital and when they leave the hospital. "Success in my mind," he says, "is defined as a person—a child, for example—who grows and you see them develop into a new person whose skills may be modified, but who is still the same inner person. Amazingly, that person has overcome tremendous physical and maybe emotional problems to go on and lead a productive life. With children, it is most gratifying because of the long follow-up period. At Shriners, they get good follow-up care because they know they are getting the best possible care without a financial hardship. It's been my experience since I came to Cincinnati in 1988, that after seeing a child for seven or eight years, you really get to see the progress they have made. You look back and say, 'Boy, I didn't think that kid would survive and look at him now. He's in high school or he's in sixth grade.' Our teenagers, many of whom return until they are 21 and have their last appointment, are sometimes married, always happy, have a family and sometimes children. That is success!"

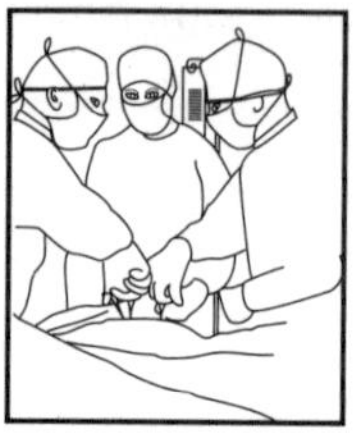

23

Ryan Zinn: New heart, new beginning

It was 1987. Ryan Zinn had gone through 14 years of perfect health. He was active, played several sports, always in nonstop motion. He attended Tiffin High School in Tiffin, Ohio, near the Ohio/West Virginia border. Late fall. Football season had just ended. "Things were going pretty well I thought," says Zinn. "I had a good football season and was getting ready for basketball. I was 14. It was my freshman year. My brother was a senior. One day at basketball practice we were running suicides, back and forth on the court. I was doing my sprints and all of a sudden things got suddenly quiet and everything faded out to black. I could still run. In fact, I was running full speed down the court but I couldn't hear a thing. Couldn't see a thing. I could feel the vibration from the runners next to me. But something was definitely wrong. So I just stopped and sat down in the bleachers. At that point, my coach said I should go to the doctor and find out what's wrong."

The doctor diagnosed Zinn as having the flu or sports asthma. He was looking for answers. He got none. "I just kind of laid low through Christmas. On December 26, I entered the hospital with heart palpitations," recalls Zinn vividly. That set off a seven-week hospitalization in January and February 1988. I went from the Medical College of Toledo to my own hospital in Tiffin to the Cleveland Clinic." Again, no one could give Zinn any answers.

Finally, doctors at the Cleveland Clinic had an answer. "Ryan," they said, "we don't know what happened, but we know what the result is. You have an enlarged heart. It's about the size of a football minus the ends. You really can't do anything. You have to walk through life if you are going to stay in this condition. You can either try a heart transplant or you can take some drugs and wait it out."

At that point, there was not much media attention about transplantation. There was no information readily available to the general public according to Zinn. "So we said 'yes' to the drug therapy. We would wait it out. At that point I still had my brain. I had always said that I wanted to be valedictorian. I could still do that. I could still reach that goal but I would just have to walk through life. I could accept that. I figured that's good enough for me. I'll be with my family and I can survive. We did this through the end of my freshman year. I turned 15 in May."

At the end of Zinn's freshman year he started to go into congestive heart failure. He had trouble eating the entire summer. "I couldn't do a thing," says Zinn. "It got to the point where I was so tired lying on the couch that my mom would walk by and think I was sleeping. But I would say to her, 'Mom, I'm just too tired. I can't even open my eyes.' It was a terrible experience that lead into drug-induced hepatitis because of all the medicine I was taking. I wasn't getting any results."

During the second week of classes in Zinn's sophomore year, he was doing his geometry homework. "I could feel myself having a stroke," recalls Zinn. "My left arm was going everywhere. I had no control over what was going on. I yelled to my mom. Obviously I could understand what I was saying in my brain, but she was hearing a big garbled mess of sounds. She knew what it was thank goodness. And she got me to the hospital. After being rushed to the Cleveland Clinic by ambulance, I met with my doctor after he had run some tests.

He said, "Ryan, you've got six months to live. What are you going to do?"

"Not much choice, really. It was a heart transplant or six months to live. Not even a second passed before I said, 'Sign me up!'"

Zinn was diagnosed with idiopathic congestive cardiomyopathy, a disease of the heart muscle. Idiopathic means they are not sure what caused it. The doctors think it was an unknown viral infection. "It could have been I caught it from a friend of mine who had mononucleosis that I got too close to," admits Zinn matter-of-factly. "Or it could have been from an over-the-counter drug that affected me beyond what it would do to someone else.

"It's nonstop. You have to be aware of your body and all the things around you. It's a never-ending process, a never-ending story. But I think that kind of helps us. It keeps us aware. I know my body better than anyone around me, other than other transplant recipients. We know our bodies, and that's good I think because we're more in tune. I think we have a better chance."

I ask Zinn if he was ever afraid of dying, relating to him that I felt so bad at times I wished I were dead. It was an existence, not really living.

"All through my nine months of sickness leading to the transplant, I don't really remember ever saying to my parents that I wished I was dead. I never remembered that because that meant giving up and I just wouldn't let myself do that. There were many times when I would ask, 'Why me?' Everybody asks 'Why me?' I never really got the answer. But I never ever wished that my life would end. If anything, I prayed to get better. I always hoped I would get better. And really, after the stroke, I realized that I was kidding myself. There was only one thing to do. When my doctor said six months to live, I thought well, you know, what can I do in six months? I'd have Thanksgiving and Christmas. Had I realized in that split second when I'm thinking of how far I could get, I thought you're crazy, you're stupid. You're not gonna let this go. You're not going to do this to your family or yourself or your friends. You're going to fight. So I did!"

Zinn received his new heart on September 26, 1988, at the Cleveland Clinic. He was in the hospital 12 days before being released. During those 12 days he had three seizures because his new heart was so powerful. "My body was in shock because my blood was pumping so fast," he relates. The doctors and nurses were actually kind of excited about the seizures because to them that indicated the heart was working well. "I was freaked out," says Zinn without hesitation. "I was a little nervous but the heart team thought it was a really good sign. Once I got past the pain of the chest opening I really noticed a big difference. My muscles were sore for the first couple of days. But I could tell things were a little better, slowly but surely."

Zinn had lost a lot of weight, going from 150 to 115 pounds. He lost muscle mass. "I wasn't to the point where I couldn't move at all but I couldn't go out and walk a good distance before the transplant. Right after the transplant, I still didn't have muscle mass but I could feel it coming back inside."

The day after he was released from the hospital, Zinn was back in school. "I went for a hour to see some friends and talk to my teachers," says Zinn. "I wanted to kind of get back in the groove. The next day I was there for about two hours. Each day I stayed a little longer and within two weeks I was back to my full schedule. At that point, because of a pull-push thing with my sternum being sawed and broken, I had to let it heal. I had someone to carry my books for a while, but other than that everything was relatively normal.

That spring, Zinn returned for track and field competition. "After waiting the required six weeks," says Zinn, "the doctors said I could basically do anything I wanted. That same day I was back in the weight room because I wanted to run again."

Zinn decided against playing football but in hindsight regrets his decision. "If I had it to do over again I would have been playing football as soon as they cleared me." Zinn says the doctor was not so concerned with the chest contact but rather about the consequences of a compound fracture and infection. The doctor said in essence his sternum was going to be stronger after the transplant than it was before. "But he warned me about breaking a leg and the possible infection. In 1988, not a lot of information or studies had been done to confirm or deny this."

At that point, Zinn began to look up to another heart transplant recipient from the Cleveland Clinic named Jeff Swanson. Swanson, from

Mentor, Ohio, was 10 years old when he was transplanted and began taking soccer balls off his chest and participating in other athletic activities that scared his doctors "silly" as Zinn says. "He pushed and he persevered," says Zinn, "and I thought, hey, if he can do it, I can do it. My one regret is that I didn't push to play football again. I wish that I would have."

When I ask him if it bothers him that his life span is going to be shorter than most people his age, Zinn says a couple of things cross his mind. "When I was in high school, I had so many goals that it seemed like I didn't have any time to die. I wasn't worried about dying. As the years went on, and it got past four years, that was a halfway point for me. I started thinking things like I don't know if I'm going to have kids. I don't even know if I'm going to have grandkids. I don't even know if I'm going to be around to retire. And it kind of struck me. It was very uncomfortable because I'm working as hard as I can to get the best education so I can get the best job. You know, to make money and have a secure future. But I don't know what the future will be. It was unsettling to me. I never thought about dying when I was sick, but now that I'm perfectly healthy I think about it more often. And I think am I questioning myself too much? You know, am I going to die because I'm making myself sick worrying about the education or the job? Or should I just live day by day? Or should I have more fun because I don't know if I'm going to be here? And as I ask more and more questions, I realize that it doesn't matter. I just need to live like I'm going to be here for another 50 years because, well I don't know, maybe I will."

Zinn's mindset has changed on how he views life since the transplant. "I was always a little more mature than my peers before the transplant," says Zinn. "I always appreciated things a little more. Maybe I was a little more serious than my friends. But certainly after the transplant I've appreciated life a lot more. I notice the little things that matter more. With them, just going out and partying and having a good time were all they needed in life in high school. I liked that too I have to admit. Usually I was the designated driver because I didn't drink. Then I realized that there is nothing more important than family. I'm going to take care of my family before I ever consider taking care of anything else."

Zinn's donor was in a car accident outside Cleveland. It was covered in the newspapers. Zinn was in the Cleveland Clinic at the time being given an I.V. to kick-start his heart a little bit, to give him more time. "It just happened that before I left the hospital, the crash occurred. The doctors told me to get ready. So we saw the news in the paper and put two and two together. I've never had personal contact with the family. My mother has sent a couple of letters and we've had a couple sent to us and it has been a good relationship. Neither family is pushing to make it an issue. I do know he was 21, relatively young like myself. I was 15. But they are happy just to know I'm doing well and that I'm carrying on his life I guess. That makes it easier."

Zinn says he doesn't think about his donor every day. His mother had contact with the family in 1995 and he asked her not to tell him his name. "I wanted to know him as the guy who gave me life," he says. "And I know everything. I know he was an ROTC student and I know he was a very good college student. He was 21, athletic, and an all-around good guy. He was a person everybody wanted to be around. I thank God I had the opportunity to get the transplant."

Zinn says he takes things one day at a time, setting goals and trying hard to reach those goals. "You can dream. You know you can't do it all in one day but you try and do everything you can every day. It is what we do with the challenges that make all the difference. A family reached out to me with love and humanity by donating their son's heart. All my pain and struggling back to the normal life of a teenager was easy compared to theirs, and I will be forever grateful. They are the true heroes.

"It certainly wasn't easy to overcome the effects of the stroke and to regain my physical endurance, but I was determined to reach out in pursuit of my dreams. I had been leading my class academically and was an avid athlete, so there was much work to be done. With the aid of a tutor and many hours spent in the weight room, I reached that dream of becoming valedictorian and even helped my track 4 x 100 meter relay team break a school record. I concentrated on what I could do and tried not to think about what I could not do. Transplantation has made me a better person. I look at everything differently and realize that with determination and desire I can meet the toughest of challenges."

Zinn has played hard in the U.S. Transplant Games. He participated in the 1992 games in Los Angeles, the 1994 games in Atlanta, the 1996 games in Salt Lake City, the 1998 games at Ohio State University in Columbus, Ohio, where he was named "Outstanding Male Athlete of the Games," and the 2000 games at Disney World's Wide World of Sports complex in Orlando. Since 1994, Zinn has won his share of medals. But more than medals, Zinn takes pride in the fact that he can help promote organ and tissue donor awareness to the public, whether it's speaking to groups or getting the media involved.

On June 8, 1996, Zinn carried the Olympic torch as it made its way to Atlanta. He was one of the 2,500 "local heroes" selected by Coca-Cola who helped carry the torch on its 15,000-mile cross-country trek.

Currently, Zinn is a process engineer with Metatec International in Dublin, Ohio. He received a master of science degree in industrial and systems engineering and manufacturing. His future plans for the next 5 years include obtaining his professional engineer (PE) certificate for Ohio and an MBA from Ohio State.

Zinn is also a track coach at Worthington Kilbourne High School in Worthington, Ohio, outside Columbus. He also has purchased a house in Worthington.

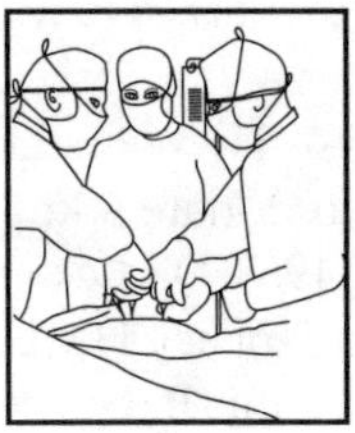

24

Dave Browe's two "gifts of life"

Dave Browe had his first kidney transplant when he was 18 and a senior at Saint Xavier High School in Cincinnati. He was among the first kidney transplant recipients at Children's Hospital Medical Center (CHMC). CHMC began its kidney transplant program in 1965.

Dialysis was cumbersome. "It was done in the hospital," remembers Browe, whose was born with a diseased kidney. "After dialysis, my system was cleansed but I always knew when it was time again because my system would slow down. I was always cold and tired. My creatinine was so high that my kidney wasn't functioning at all."

Browe's family – three brothers and two sisters – moved to Cincinnati from Chicago in 1967, where Browe began as a senior at Saint Xavier High School. "I met some really nice guys where we lived," recalls Browe. "I started carpooling with them. But by October I began to feel miserable. By November, things were really going downhill. Cincinnati Bell, the local telephone company, came out to our house and put in a speaker that was connected to my room. Another student was designated to carry the box to my classes." His attempt at home schooling didn't work and Browe graduated a year later at Saint Xavier. "The school made every effort to keep me going through senior year. It just didn't work out."

Browe's friends at Saint Xavier and Roger Bacon High School knew he was in serious condition. Browe himself knew it better than anyone. "At one point," says Browe, "I was sure I was going to die. Maybe 'sure' is the wrong word. I was fairly certain it was going to be a 50-50 shot. I did write out a will, just to have something. I mean, what have you got at 18. You've got $300 in the bank and some books or whatever. But I did write it out and give it to my folks."

Browe says his parents, to their credit, tried to keep things as normal as possible. His older sister, Penny, now a nurse, had just started at Northern Kentucky University. "Penny was aware of my condition and that there was extra pressure on her taking care of my younger brothers and sisters who were 12, 10, 6, and 5.

That year, 1967, Browe was in and out of CHMC, usually for about two to three weeks at a time. "There'd be nights when all of a sudden mom and dad would come down to see me at the hospital and they didn't come home for a while, if things were going bad."

Browe was released from CHMC for Christmas in 1967. He knew he was going to have a kidney transplant. "Mom was going to donate a kidney," recalls Browe. The transplant took place on January 15, 1968. Dr. Lester Martin and Dr. Luis L. Gonzalez performed the kidney transplant at CHMC.

The surgery was complicated. Browe's urologist, Dr. John Babcock, was called in because of excess scar tissue from the dialysis. The operation lasted 11 hours. Browe remained in isolation for 11 days. After 10 more days in the hospital, he was allowed to go home.

After being home for six weeks, Browe suffered a major rejection. This time, he stayed in CHMC for six weeks. Browe was taking prednisone and azathioprine for immunosuppression. "I was taking massive doses of prednisone. One reason I had to stay in the hospital so long was because the prednisone gave me an ulcer."

Browe says at age 18 his biggest concern was the puffiness in his face that occurred with the prednisone. "The *Cincinnati Enquirer* took a picture of the first eight of us that had kidney transplants at CHMC. I was propped up in the back because I was still in the hospital when they took the photo. In the caption, it said that 'the puffiness that appears in these children will eventually disappear. It is because of the high doses of medication they're taking.' My biggest problem at the time was not a big problem. And it sounds like vanity more than anything else. I'm going through my teenage years and I've got a little interest in the girls on the one hand and I'm trying to be macho and you're sitting there looking like hell and feeling like hell on the other end. My face just puffed up. I'm sitting there saying to myself, 'God, look in the mirror. I look like the man in the moon only redder.'"

Browe's first kidney lasted 14 years. His clinic visits that first year were frequent. He graduated from Saint Xavier in 1969. When he was looking into colleges to attend, the doctors at CHMC preferred he be no more than one hour away from the hospital. "I ended up going to the University of Dayton (UD)," he says. "I liked the school, it worked out great, and I was close enough to CHMC. My freshman year at UD I was coming to CHMC once a month."

Browe is the first to admit he's always had a little problem remembering to take his medicine. He and I were manning an organ and tissue donation display a few years ago at the Butler County Fair when he told me about forgetting to take his medicine. "The first time I ever heard the word non-compliant was from you," he tells me.

Three days later he went into The Christ Hospital where he now has his follow-up work done. "They asked me how often I took a particular medication and I said, 'Well . . . you know.'"

"So you're non-compliant, huh?"

"In 32 years I had never heard the word non-compliant," says Browe. "And in one week I heard it twice. Non-compliant to me suggests that you sit down and decide you're not going to take your medicine. I've gotten into sloppy habits. I've discussed this with my nephrologist, Dr. Nina Mendoza, and transplant surgeon Dr. Wes Alexander. Dr. Alexander used to look at me and shake his head and say, 'Gee, I don't know how you do it.' I don't take my medication on a daily basis, but I don't get up in the morning and say I'm not taking my medicine. I've just gotten in the habit where I forget. You say, 'Okay, how can I forget when you open the medicine cabinet and there's all the medication.' Well, I get busy shaving and somebody wants this and somebody wants that. I mean on a weekly basis, to be totally honest, five out of seven days is good. I'm happy with that."

Browe is convinced that he has built up his own special immune system. "I don't get sick that often. I feel I'm healthy all the time. I figured out once that I've taken almost 100,000 pills since my transplant."

Browe studied liberal arts at the University of Dayton. He met his wife, Jill, in 1969, at the end of his senior year at Saint Xavier. "We met on a blind date," recalls Browe. "I started dating her that summer and then went off to college and we kept dating." Browe graduated in April 1973 and they were married in June 1973. They have three daughters. Robin is in college. Betsy and Ellen are in high school.

By 1982, Browe needed another kidney transplant. The serious rejection episode he suffered in 1968 caused the reduction of his kidney function. This time, Browe's younger brother, Mark, donated one of his kidneys. He received the transplant in June 1982 at The Christ Hospital. "The whole family offered to be the donor," says Browe. "It worked out that Mark was the best match."

Browe says faith played a key role in his survival. "I have a great appreciation for life. After 32 years as a transplant recipient I have experienced all the love, dedication, and sacrifice of those who are part of the transplant process—family, organ donors, and medical professionals. The words organ donor and courage are synonymous in my mind, for whether it is a living donor or a cadaver, people have made an unselfish choice motivated by love. You really have to have faith through the whole thing. You have to believe that for one reason or another there is a purpose."

Browe has always liked athletics, as both a participant and a spectator. In 1990, 1992, 1994, and 1996, he competed in the U.S. Transplant Games. Browe won a bronze medal in badminton at the 1992 games in Los Angeles. He won a gold medal in badminton at the 1994 games in Atlanta. At the 1996 games in Salt Lake City, he won a bronze medal in badminton. And in

1998 games at Ohio State University, he won a gold in badminton. "I've enjoyed the camaraderie of the games," says Browe. "It's a real nice way of getting together with people who have a common interest and something in common. It is a real sense of sharing with people." He participated in the 2000 U.S. Transplant Games at Disney World in Orlando, June 21–24.

Currently, Browe is a real estate agent and has a consulting business on the Web. His wife, Jill, is a nurse at The Christ Hospital in Cincinnati where she teaches phlebotomy.

The use of prednisone over a 32-year period has taken its toll on Browe. "My hips and knees are being affected. Dr. Mendoza has suggested I have knee replacements but I'm not interested in doing that at this point. I can still walk and run. As I tell people, I don't do either one well but I can still do them. As long as I can do it and tolerate the pain, then I'm going to keep it that way." In October 1998 Browe had one of his hips replaced. The surgery went well and he recovered with the help of excellent physical therapy.

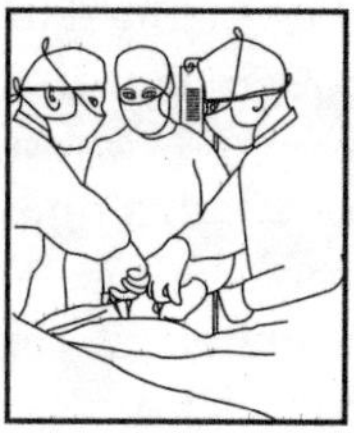

25

Corneal recipient is seeing stars again

(Author's note: The following chapter was written by Theresa Eisenburg, former education coordinator, of the Cincinnati Eye Bank.)

A nighttime sky filled with twinkling starts is so universal that the subject is portrayed in nursery rhymes and children's songs. We wish upon the stars to ensure that our dreams come true. For Dr. David Mehringer, medical science and his own hard work have enabled him to fulfill his dream of becoming an astronomer.

Since birth, Mehringer has suffered with a variety of eyesight problems and has undergone more than 20 ophthalmic operations. Two of the surgeries were corneal transplants to enhance his vision. Mehringer was born with glaucoma, which is relatively rare in infants and children. It is a condition of high pressure within the eye and requires medical treatment. Mehringer also had cataracts. Most often associated with older adults, cataracts involve the lens of the eye. The natural lens loses it clarity and is surgically removed. It is usually replaced with a tiny, lightweight plastic disk known as an intraocular lens. Mehringer also was born very myopic, or nearsighted, and could not see objects far away.

He describes his eyesight before any of his surgeries as "very, very bad." The score for normal vision is 20/20, meaning a person standing 20 feet away from an eye chart can read what the average person can at that distance. "I couldn't even see the *E* on the eye chart," admits Mehringer, who scored 20/500 on the vision test, a result 25 times worse than normal.

Eye surgery compensated for some of Mehringer's vision problems. He had his first corneal transplant at 14 in 1979. Dr. Arden Wander at University Hospital in Cincinnati removed the defective cornea in Mehringer's left eye and replaced it with a healthy donor cornea.

Mehringer graduated from Cincinnati's Deer Park High School and then began college at Denison University in central Ohio to study physics. By this time, his sight had deteriorated and he could not see well enough, even with corrective lenses, to read. In order to complete his course assignments, Mehringer hauled notes, handouts, and books across campus where he used a closed-circuit television to magnify the printed materials up to 60 times.

Mehringer decided he needed to be able to see better if he planned to pursue a career in astronomy. At 21, he convinced Dr. Wander to perform a second corneal transplant. The Cincinnati Eye Bank recovered a cornea from a 16-year-old donor and once again Dr. Wander operated, this time on David's right eye.

The corneal transplant enhanced Mehringer's sight tremendously. He could enjoy reading again, not only textbooks and journal articles associated with his pursuit of a bachelor's degree, but also printed materials for pleasure. A fan of science fiction and fantasy, he admits to spending more than a few hours browsing through bookstores and always visits Barnes and Noble when he returns to Cincinnati. These visits to his hometown once or twice a year also permit him to spend time with family and friends.

Mehringer also has enjoyed unexpected benefits from his corneal transplants. "I win a lot more at chess than I did," he laughingly confesses. Prior to his second corneal transplant, he could not make out the pieces on the board and had to memorize where each piece landed after every move. Although his chess partner is not pleased with his increased success at the game, Mehringer admits he still fails to emerge victorious from every match. The same holds true regarding his proficiency with a pool cue. As he says, "Now the balls actually go in the pockets."

Perhaps the most poignant aspect of the second corneal transplant, however, concerns Mehringer's fascination with the universe. Remembering childhood nights spent gazing into the skies, he reveals, "After the corneal transplant, I could see the stars again. That's very inspirational to me and it's what motivated me to become an astronomer in the first place."

Mehringer continued his work in physics after graduating from Denison University in 1988. He attended the University of Chicago, obtaining both his M.S. and Ph.D. in astrophysics. Currently a post-doctoral scholar at the California Institute of Technology in Pasadena, he faces quite a commute some days, traveling from southern California to the Big Island of Hawaii. Once there, he rides with fellow astronomers in a four-wheel drive vehicle along narrow, winding roads to the top of Mauna Kea, a dormant volcano. Perched 14,000 feet above sea level in Caltech's Submillimeter Observatory, Mehringer studies the chemistry of stellar nurseries, regions in which solar systems similar to ours may be forming. These studies provide important insights into the complexity of the chemistry in our solar system in its beginning.

While it sounds enticing to work in Hawaii, he confesses the reality is not quite as glamorous. Because of the high altitude, the air is so thin that breathing is labored and the nights so cold a parka is required. The nature of his work—since stars obviously appear after the sun sets—requires Mehringer and his colleagues to stay up all night, then sleep during the day. He concedes there is little spare time to visit the beach.

While leading a team of scientists as a post-doctoral fellow at the University of Illinois at Urbana-Champaign, Mehringer and his colleagues detected vinegar in outer space. Vinegar, when combined with ammonia (a gas present in outer space), produces the simplest amino acid, glygine, which is one of the building blocks of life. In other words, this discovery provided additional scientific evidence regarding the possibility of the existence of extraterrestrial life.

Although Mehringer still has "obvious" vision problems, he appreciates his increased ability to see. Corneal transplants are the most common and successful of all transplant operations; however, they cannot cure all forms of blindness. In his case, the transplants eliminated the problems with his corneal blindness and enabled him to see well enough to read. He still suffers from tunnel vision—a drastic reduction of his peripheral sight—due to optic nerve damage resulting from his glaucoma. He also wears bifocals at the relatively young age of 34.

Despite his continuing vision problems, severe enough that he cannot obtain a driver's license, Mehringer nevertheless is "very appreciative" that his vision is much improved as a result of the transplants. He acknowledges the donor family, stating, I am very grateful for the family which had the presence of mind during a very difficult time to donate." Firm in his belief that eye, tissue, and organ donation is "very important," he intends to become a donor and would encourage others to donate as well. "It's a way for loved ones to live on in someone else and is one of the greatest gifts someone could give."

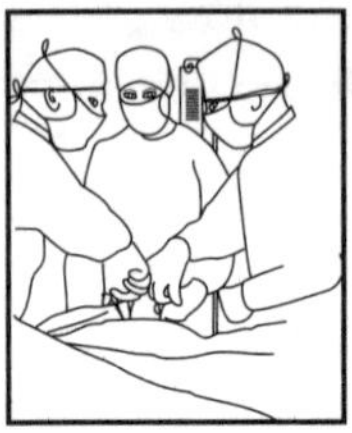

26

Freedom from dialysis has special meaning for kidney transplant recipients

"July 10, 2000, marked the four-year anniversary of my third and most successful kidney transplant," says Theo Smith of Mount Airy, a Cincinnati suburb. Smith had a living-related transplant in 1988 from his brother in Miami, Florida, and two cadaver transplants from The Christ Hospital in 1992 and July 10, 1996. Today, he is doing well and has returned to work as community education specialist for LifeCenter. "Daily, what comes to mind is the sheer feeling of freedom from hemodialysis, I'm sure the same unparalleled, healthy feeling that flowers share when basking in the sun, growing more lively and vital each day, rain or shine. Getting back the 12 to 15 hours a week I lost while on dialysis has enabled me more quality time with my wife, children, and friends."

Dialysis, both hemodialysis and peritoneal, removes toxins and waste products of metabolism, and fluid from a patient's blood, doing the work of the kidneys. It can be both physically and mentally exhausting. If disease or trauma damage a patient's kidneys, dialysis or a kidney transplant are the only options. Dialysis keeps some of these patients with end-stage renal disease (ESRD) alive. Many are on waiting lists for a kidney transplant or they may get one from a living donor, such as a relative or spouse. Nausea, vomiting, and weakness are common side effects of dialysis.

"With hemodialysis, the blood is circulated through a computer-controlled dialysis machine," says Dr. Roy First, director of transplant nephrology at University Hospital in Cincinnati. "A needle is inserted into the patient's arm to draw the blood out through the machine which takes out all the toxins. It then returns the patient's blood through a second needle in the patient's arm." The surgical joining of an artery and a vein in the patient's arm, called a fistula, provides the needed access for these needles. A patient spends three or four hours three times week for hemodialysis.

"Peritoneal dialysis utilizes the peritoneum or lining of the bowel around the abdominal cavity," says Dr. First. "A catheter is inserted firmly into the abdominal cavity. Fluid runs into this cavity for a period of 30 minutes to six hours with chronic ambulatory peritoneal dialysis (CAPD) or eight to 10 hours per night with continuous peritoneal dialysis (CPD). With CPD, the patient is hooked up to an automated machine that completes the dialysis in more rapid cycles. There are usually three or four exchanges a day with CAPD. With peritoneal dialysis, the fluid comes in contact with the peritoneum, which has a very rich blood supply, and the waste products and toxins come out of the blood in the peritoneal fluid. That fluid is discarded."

A patient on peritoneal dialysis may require more exchanges each day than a patient on hemodialysis, but peritoneal dialysis is somewhat portable, giving patients greater mobility.

"Either form of dialysis (hemodialysis or peritoneal dialysis) is very variable according to the individual," says Dr. First. Each person is different. Some patients don't want to consider a transplant. They may be doing well on dialysis. Dialysis does take its toll, though, over the years. You see gradual deterioration in a patient's overall well-being. You have to speak to patients who have been on dialysis and then had a successful transplant in order to assess the differences in emotion and stress. It varies largely according to the individual."

Lori Gebell-Dalby of Clermont County, east of Cincinnati, developed kidney disease while in grade school. She had chronic glomerulonephritis, an inflammation of the glomeruli of the kidney and was treated by physicians at Children's Hospital Medical Center (CHMC). She was put on peritoneal dialysis for four to five months, 16 hours per day. This grueling schedule made her practically confined to dialysis treatment. After this, she was maintained on medications such as diuretics for about nine months. While this was better than being on dialysis, her condition deteriorated. For the next year and a half she was on hemodialysis, three days a week, four hours a day. "It seems like I just had to wait to get worse," says Dalby. "I remember the needle sticks with bore cannula needles. I was a child with a chronic disease. I was disturbed by all the terminology the doctors at Children's Hospital were using. I had constant doctors' appointments, had to be tutored for school, and felt worse than someone with chronic fatigue syndrome. I did feel good about a day after the hemodialysis treatment, but my lifestyle was largely that of being strapped to a machine. I went to school on my off days from dialysis."

Dalby received a kidney transplant on October 5, 1980, at CHMC. She was 13 years old and was in the seventh grade. "At 13, I was a little apprehensive at first about the transplant, but since I've had it I've never looked back," she says. "I was hesitant about my medications after the transplant. I saw other kids who had puffy cheeks and moon faces. I had no idea how they felt, only how they looked to me. But after my transplant I felt wonderful. I'm very conscious of my health and probably go to extremes to maintain it. I view dialysis as a bridge that was necessary to keep me alive, although it was a very emotional bridge. I have heard and read that ESRD is one of the most depressing diseases, affecting patients both physically and emotionally." In 20 years Dalby has had no rejection of her kidney.

Today, Dalby is 33 and an operating room (OR) nurse at Bethesda North Hospital. She graduated from Bethesda's nursing program. "Growing up with a kidney transplant, I was my own patient advocate," admits Dalby. She continues to promote organ and tissue donation among her hospital colleagues and the general public. Dalby was married in October 1995, close to her transplant anniversary.

"As an OR nurse at Bethesda North, I have been involved with several organ recoveries with LifeCenter. While I mourn for the donor and donor family, I rejoice for the recipients," she says tearfully.

Dalby knows very little about her donor, only that he was a 23-year-old male from Miami, Florida. She thinks about him often and prays for his family.

Dr. First says a kidney transplant will, in the first few months, have "a slightly higher mortality rate than dialysis. But the transplant then has very good long-term survival rates. In dialysis, there is a constant loss of life year by year. People on dialysis for 10 or 15 years experience side effects like bone deterioration, anemia, and sexual dysfunction."

In 1998, Medicare's budget for ESRD reached $14.5 billion. Of this, $13.5 billion was paid for dialysis, while $1 to $2 billion went to pay for kidney transplantation. "The vast majority of this money is spent on dialysis," says Dr. First. "There are more than 300,000 patients on dialysis in the United States, roughly 250,000 of those on Medicare. More than forty-six thousand people are waiting for kidney transplants in the United States while more than 145 are waiting in Greater Cincinnati. The cost for one year of dialysis is about $40,000 to $45,000. A kidney transplant costs about $80,000 for the first year, including follow-up tests and immunosuppressive medications. But after that first year, patient cost is about $6,000 per year. Dialysis is still $45,000 per year. In three to five years, transplantation is far more cost effective. However, if a kidney transplant fails, it is more costly for the patient and the healthcare system. Fortunately, unlike other organ transplants, kidney patients can return to dialysis."

Dr. First says a major impetus to kidney transplantation is a discrepancy with healthcare insurance companies. Many private insurers do not have much of an incentive to have patients in their plan transplanted, especially if they are on Medicare.

"During the first 18 months of ESRD entitlement, the patient's paid group health insurance is primary for either dialysis or a kidney transplant," says Kay Bonar, an administrative assistant to Dr. First. "After this entitlement, it switches from your group health insurance to Medicare. I've had insurance companies ask me why we didn't wait until the patient reaches 18 months because they don't want to be the primary insurance for the transplant."

Says Dr. First: "If only Medicare were involved as the patient's insurer there would be a tremendous incentive to promote organ donation and transplantation."

The change in an ESRD patient after a successful kidney transplant occurs very rapidly according to Dr. First. "For successful transplant patients who were on dialysis, their overall well-being enables them to resume their lives and sometimes return to work. We would like to see more recipients gainfully employed."

Theo Smith feels this change every day. "Each time I look in the mirror, I'm reminded of how I've changed, both physically and emotionally. It is overwhelming sometimes, like the feeling of gratification and unsurpassed enjoyment I have when working in our yard at home. Above all, there is the realization of the importance and blessing organ donation and transplantation has meant to my family and me. It can drastically change lives!"

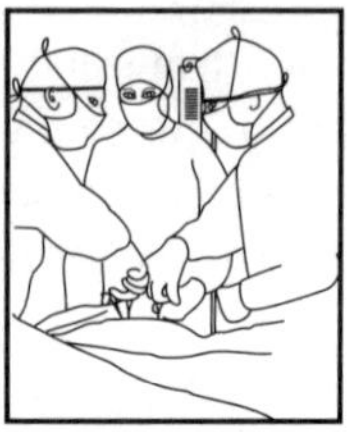

27

Heart transplant recipient runs in New York Marathon

Greg Osterman loves to run because it makes him feel good. So good in fact that he ran in the New York City Marathon on November 7, 1999. With a temperature of 42° and a windchill of 18°, Osterman finished the race in just over five hours.

He appeared briefly on NBC's *Today* show on November 6 prior to the race. Upon returning to Greater Cincinnati he appeared on WLWT-TV on November 10 and on a sports segment called *Harvey's Heroes* on WKRC-TV. There were also features in *Community Press, Inc.'s* suburban newspaper group and in the December 1999 issue of *Runner's World*, a national magazine.

But the road to feeling good was a rocky one for the 46-year-old from Loveland, Ohio, just outside of Cincinnati, who is also a certified volunteer with LifeCenter. On October 26, 1992, Osterman had a heart transplant at University Hospital in Cincinnati. Diagnosed with cardiomyopathy, a weakening of the heart muscle, doctors believed a virus was the cause. After 14 days in the hospital, Osterman headed home. "For two months or so I just took things one day at a time," says the soft-spoken Osterman. In the spring of 1993, he returned to work as a commercial plumber.

Osterman was on the track team at Cincinnati's Moeller High School. But he had never run a marathon before. After the heart transplant, he says, "I was amazed to be able to walk again. But then everything I used to take for granted came back to me and I just pushed myself a little and that progressed into running marathons."

Osterman's good health was short-lived. A routine cardiac biopsy in March 1993 indicated rejection. "I was put in the hospital and took all the necessary immunosuppressive medications for three days," recalls Osterman. "I went home but never did feel quite right. My energy level was down and I couldn't understand why. Then, for some strange reason, I don't know why, I noticed I was bleeding internally. I immediately called cardiac transplant and they ran some tests. The immunosuppressive medications had lowered my immune system and the cancer—non-Hodgkin's lymphoma—had started in my intestinal area. That's why I was bleeding. I went into University Hospital and was given a blood transfusion. The doctors thought they had the problem corrected and they were going to reduce my immunosuppressive medications. I did stop bleeding internally and was sent home. In three days, it started again. An endoscopy revealed the intestinal cancer had grown."

Osterman underwent extensive surgery to remove several parts of his small and large intestines and gall bladder. He was hospitalized during March and April 1993. Under the care of Dr. Elyse Lower at the Barrett Cancer Center, he received follow-up treatment for a year. The Barrett Center worked in conjunction with University Hospital's cardiac transplant clinic. His immunosuppressive medications were lowered to try to boost his immune system to fight off the cancer. "It was kind of touch and go for awhile," he admits. "I followed the doctors' orders to a 'T' and it all worked out."

So Osterman spent most of 1993 healing. In the fall of 1993, he was ready to begin an exercise program and returned to work as a plant engineer. "I set my sights on running in the American Heart Association's Mini-Marathon in 1994," says Osterman. "I never dreamed it would be possible. That is what got everything started. I was amazed I had come so far after everything that had happened. I set my sights on longer distances. Three years later I decided to do a marathon. I spent six months training and in 1998 I ran the Bermuda Marathon. I was the first heart transplant recipient to run the Bermuda Marathon." Osterman then ran in the San Diego Marathon and the Flying Pig Marathon in Cincinnati.

His training regimen for a marathon is usually for five months before the marathon. He runs two to three times a week for five or six miles and two 15-mile runs on the weekend. Three weeks before the marathon Osterman runs 20 miles. During this time he also lifts weights and works on upper body strength as well.

"It was pretty scary when I first started to run," says Osterman. "I didn't know if I was doing myself good or not. I didn't know if pushing myself to the limit was what the doctors intended or whether I should just get back to a normal routine. I checked with the doctors on everything I did. They told me if I felt like doing it to go ahead. They gave me signs to watch for. After a certain point you realize you can run further. You run a 5K and say, 'I feel pretty good. I bet I could do a 10K.' You run a 10K and don't feel bad and say, 'I'll do a 15K.' It feels great to be able to do it."

Osterman runs year-round until it gets to be 10° or colder. He says today's running clothes keep you fairly comfortable. "I enjoy running in snow. It's great. It takes your mind totally off running."

Throughout his ordeal, the support of Osterman's family—his wife, Carol, and sons Jason and Danny—contributed greatly to his success. "My family went through this with me," he says. "I can't say enough about my wife. I was sick for two years with another year of recuperation. She took care of the house, the bills, the kids, everything, in addition to working."

Says wife Carol: "I think the hardest part of hearing about Greg's diagnosis and prospect for the future was hearing the bottom line. His only hope for survival was a heart transplant. Greg and I just looked at each other, unable to comment to the doctors. We were in shock. In 1990, a transplant was still rare—a big risk. I felt nervous, helpless, lost. That was such an extreme treatment for Greg's problem. I thought of our two children and what the future would bring for all of us. It seemed hopeless to me. I assumed that even if Greg did survive the transplant, he would have a very limited quality of life. It's obvious now that I was badly mistaken and I'm very thankful.

"Then in early 1993 when the doctors found that Greg had severe intestinal bleeding, they quickly operated finding non-Hodgkin's lymphoma. The doctor's talk after the operation left me numb. His outlook for Greg seemed bleak. After everything that all of us had been through with Greg's transplant, this seemed cruel. While driving home that night, something told me that if Greg could beat his heart problem, he could also beat this. It has been more than eight years since that night. I'm still crossing my fingers and saying a prayer that I was right. We live day to day and are very grateful!"

Running not only makes Osterman feel good. It also lets other transplant recipients see that they too can get back on their feet and have an extremely good quality of life. "The more confidence you have the better your attitude will be," reasons Osterman. He ran in the American Heart Association's Cincinnati Mini-Marathon, a 10K race, in March 2000 and also participated in the U.S. Transplant Games in 2000 at Disney World in Orlando.

Section IV

Conclusion and Final Thoughts

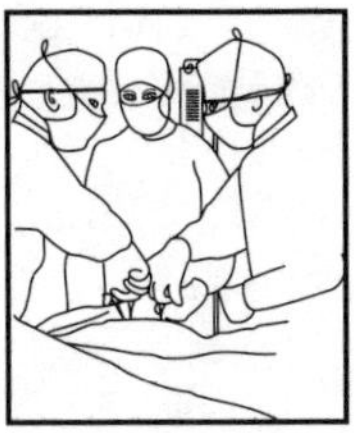

28

Working for an organ procurement organization (OPO)

When I had my heart transplant in 1989, I knew my donor was from the Greater Cincinnati area. Eventually, I met his family and we have become quite close. I knew my heart was recovered by the local organ procurement organization (OPO) Ohio Valley Organ Procurement Center, now LifeCenter, but that was about all. I did some research and found out as much about LifeCenter as I could. There are 61 other OPOs around the country that do what LifeCenter does, and that is to coordinate activities relating to organ procurement in a designated service area. In 1991, I began working for LifeCenter as an education specialist, handling public education, news releases, media coordination, and volunteer coordination. I am now public affairs manager.

I did not realize how many people were involved in the donation process: transplant surgeons; transplant coordinators on the recovery and clinical sides; the executive director of the OPO; neurosurgeons and attending physicians at the donor hospital; referring nurses from the donor hospital; hospital operating room nurses; clergy from the donor hospital; social workers from the donor hospital; the tissue typing laboratory; laboratory technicians; hospital maintenance; those handling air and ground transportation; telephone hotline coordinators; and many, many more from LifeCenter, the local, independent non-profit OPO for Greater Cincinnati individuals.

Each day in Greater Cincinnati, transplant professionals work with physicians, nurses, hospital administrators, clergy, and social workers to increase the number of life-saving organs and life-enhancing tissues available for transplantation. LifeCenter's service area includes 29 hospitals in 16 counties in southwest Ohio, northern Kentucky, and southeast Indiana: Adams, Brown, Butler, Clermont, Clinton, Hamilton, Highland, and Warren counties in Ohio; Boone, Campbell, Gallatin, Grant, Kenton and Pendleton counties in northern Kentucky; and Dearborn and Ohio counties in southeastern Indiana. LifeCenter began operating in 1981. Its service area has been approved and designated by the Health Care and Financing Administration (HCFA).

LifeCenter transplant coordinators evaluate potential organ donors, discussing the option of donation with family members of the deceased. Transplant coordinators also arrange for the surgical removal of donated organs. They preserve the organs and make arrangements for their distribution according to national organ sharing policies established by the Organ Procurement and Transplantation Network (OPTN) of the United Network for Organ Sharing (UNOS). These policies have been approved by the U.S. Department of Health and Human Services.

LifeCenter is a member of UNOS and follows all guidelines of the OPTN. LifeCenter works very closely with Ohio Valley Tissue and Skin Center (OVTSC), the Cincinnati Eye Bank, and the Midwest Ear Foundation. Through routine notification, each death at a hospital is reported to the transplant hotline for LifeCenter, OVTSC, the Cincinnati Eye Bank, and the Midwest Ear Foundation.

LifeCenter provides a 24-hour surgical and technical staff to identify, manage, recover, preserve, transport and share organs for transplantation. LifeCenter also provides professional and community education programs for healthcare professionals, schools, churches, civic, and other community organizations.

In Greater Cincinnati, there are three transplant centers. Children's Hospital Medical Center performs pediatric kidney, liver, and heart transplants. University Hospital performs kidney, kidney/pancreas, heart, and liver transplants. The Christ Hospital performs adult kidney transplants.

In the United States, there are 244 kidney transplant programs; 115 liver transplant programs; 126 pancreas transplant programs; 23 pancreas islet cell transplant programs; 37 intestine transplant programs; 141 heart transplant programs; 88 heart/lung transplant programs and 80 lung transplant programs.

All patients accepted onto a transplant program's waiting list are registered with UNOS. UNOS maintains a centralized computer network linking all OPOs and transplant centers. This computer network is accessible 24 hours a day, seven days a week, with organ placement specialists always available to answer questions.

When a donor becomes available, the transplant center or OPO accesses the UNOS computer and generates a list of patients ranked according to UNOS policies on organ allocation, generally through local, regional, and then national geographic areas as timing is crucial in organ recovery.

Organs are allocated by UNOS in a fair and equitable manner. When a patient's name is added to the national list, his or her medical profile is entered and stored in the UNOS computer. The patient is not placed on a ranked list at this time. Instead, the patient's name is added to a "pool" of patient names. When a donor becomes available, the computer ranks each patient in this pool according to medical and scientific criteria. It then generates a list of patients who most closely match the donor's characteristics.

Factors affecting ranking include tissue match, blood type, length of time on the waiting list, degree of illness, and immune status. In the case of heart, heart/lung, lung, and pancreas, the potential recipient's distance from the donor hospital is also a consideration. Each donor generates a differently ranked list of patients.

After receiving a printout of the waiting list, the LifeCenter transplant coordinator contacts a transplant team of surgeons and physicians for selection of a patient. Often, the top patient will not get the organ for one of several reasons. When a patient is selected, he or she must be available, healthy enough to undergo major surgery, and willing to be transplanted immediately. Also, laboratory tests are necessary to measure compatibility between the donor and recipient. Often, patients with high antibody levels cannot be transplanted because their immune systems would reject the organs. After a patient is selected and contacted and all testing is complete, surgery is scheduled and the transplant takes place.

The commitment of the entire hospital—administration, medical staff, and nursing staff—makes the donation process work effectively through the development and implementation of donation policies. LifeCenter transplant coordinators help form these policies.

Hospital healthcare professionals and the LifeCenter staff dramatically increase the number of organs and tissues by simply working together. This team effectively provides the needed information and emotional and spiritual support to a grieving family faced with the death of a loved one and the decision about organ and tissue donation.

Families are more likely to agree to donate if they are asked some time after they have been informed of the death or imminent death of their loved one. Decoupling allows families time to deal with their grief, and share in the feeling that despite this grief, their loved one will save many lives and enhance the lives of others.

* * * * *

Tom Craycraft retired from LifeCenter early in 2000. He had been a transplant coordinator and perfusionist with LifeCenter since 1969 when it was a hospital-based OPO. He says the early days of organ recovery were pioneering. "We just recovered kidneys then," he recalls. "It was fun. It was enjoyable. It was functional. Back then we pumped kidneys on the Belzer Pump, which was named for transplant pioneer Dr. Folkert (Fred) Belzer who died in 1995.

Dr. Belzer invented the pump that kept kidneys alive through a continuous circulation for several days. He began as a transplant surgeon at the University of California (San Francisco) and later moved to the University of Wisconsin (Madison) as chair of the department of surgery. He patented University of Wisconsin solution (UW), a perfusion fluid still used today for organs to be transplanted. "It took a lot more time and a lot more perseverance in the early days," says Craycraft of organ recovery. Today at LifeCenter, kidneys from non-heartbeating donors (donors who cardiac arrest) are pumped. But the pump is much more portable, though still used at LifeCenter's lab. "The old Belzer Pump weighed 800 pounds on wheels," says Craycraft, wincing at just the thought of its size. "Now the Waters portable module which weighs about 55 pounds is used."

Craycraft says when the cardiac transplant program began in 1985 at University Hospital it "was all new to us. We had big meetings as to what we were going to do and how we were going to do it. The time element was critical. The logistics. You had to cut it down real close, and it took a lot of teamwork and effort. But everybody pitched in. I guess we were all kind of scared because we had never recovered hearts before. It was just a monumental thing."

Craycraft has an amusing story about Dr. David Melvin who started the cardiac transplant program at University Hospital in 1985. "He got the Federal Aviation Administration (FAA) after him for cutting across the National Guard airstrip in Lexington without permission during a heart recovery. The airstrip was right next to the airport in Lexington. Our ambulance driver got lost. So we ended up on the National Guard side. The driver said we'd have to go around. Dr. Melvin said, 'No, just cut straight across. I can see our plane right over there.' The guy said, 'I can't.' And Dr. Melvin said, 'You do it, this is an emergency.' We got about halfway across and boy, here come these MPs after us with their lights flashing. They caught our ass. He said, 'I'm Dr. Melvin. You can write me up or tell whomever you want to. Send me a letter when I get back to Cincinnati. We'll talk about it then. I've got a heart here to take care of first.'"

Dr. Melvin still recovers hearts for LifeCenter and assists with heart transplants. Craycraft says he's mellowed quite a bit "but still gets a little antsy. You have to realize time is still critical with the heart. The heart is the easiest organ to recover but it's also the most sensitive."

Craycraft handled a lot of paperwork for UNOS, mainly on kidney recoveries. "You have to have a good scientific background or data pool, but the paperwork gets a little overwhelming after awhile because you have periodic follow-ups plus initiating the forms and that's just for kidneys."

Craycraft has moved to Florida for retirement.

For more information about organ and tissue donation, contact the United Network for Organ Sharing (UNOS) at (804) 330-8500 or the Coalition on Donation at (800) 355-SHARE. Visit the UNOS web site at www.unos.org.

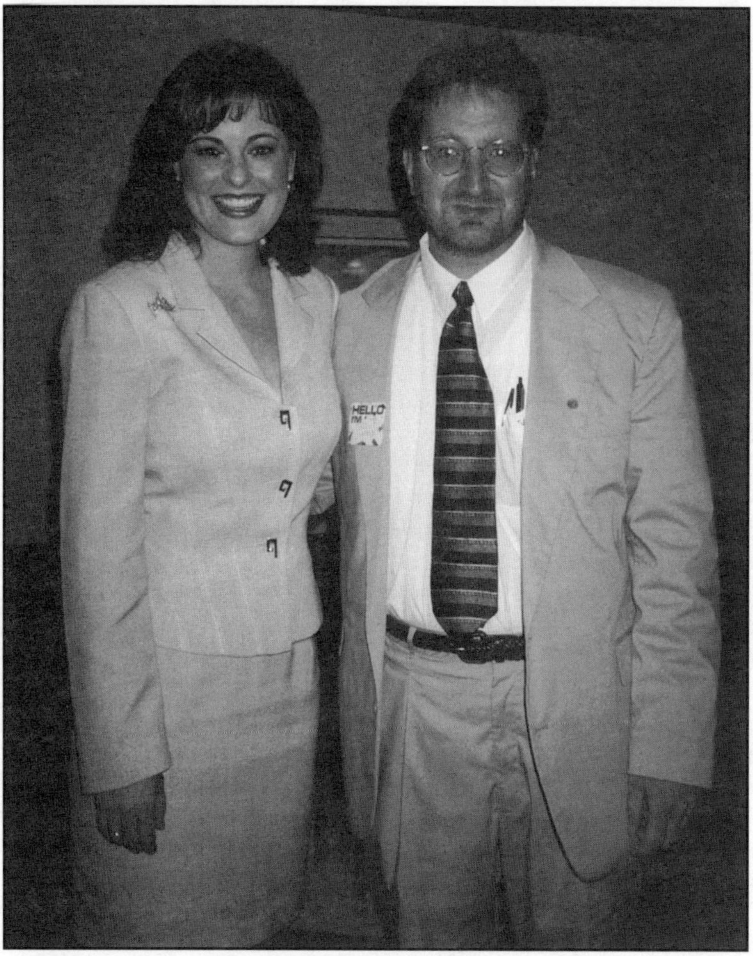

Meeting Miss America

Nicole Johnson, Miss America 1999, and Jeff Lueders at the 20th anniversary of the kidney/pancreas transplant program at Cincinnati's University Hospital. Johnson, a diabetic, has a special interest in pancreas transplantation. She wears an insulin pump for her daily insulin dosages.

Photograph © by Debbie Lueders

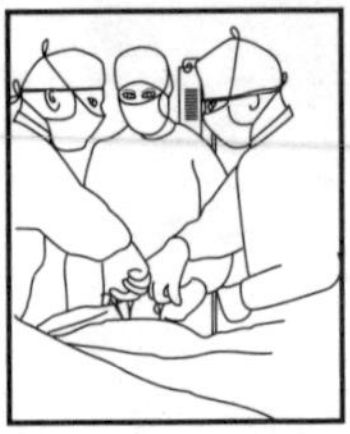

29

The need for organ and tissue donation

The need for organ and tissue donation is constantly rising. The national waiting list for organ transplants rises at a rate of more than 1,000 additional new names a month. As of October 2000, there are more than 72,000 names on the national waiting list. More than 270 wait in Greater Cincinnati alone.

On average each day in the United States, 11 men, women, children, or teenagers die because an organ is not available. Each year in the United States, 450,000 to 500,000 individuals receive a tissue transplant, 33,000 of these being corneal transplants.

Advances in healthcare and medicine, and a decrease in traumatic deaths by automobile and work-related accidents, mean that fewer and fewer organs and tissues are available for transplant.

Family members will be asked to provide consent for donation to occur. Research has shown that if family members don't know that their loved one wanted to become a donor, they may deny consent. This adds to the tragedy considering that one organ donor can save as many as eight lives, and tissue donors can save and improve the quality of life for dozens more. Donor families know their loved one is living on in others. This is the only positive aspect to emerge from a senseless tragedy.

Signing and carrying a donor card is only the first step. You need to *donate life* and share your decision with your family. Time and again, when confronted with this decision, families have said that it would have been a much easier decision to make had they known what their loved one wanted them to do.

The only way to be sure your family members do know what you want them to do in the event of your death is to tell them.

If you sign a donor card, ask your family to witness your signature. Then, encourage a family member to also consider becoming a donor and offer to witness them signing their own card.

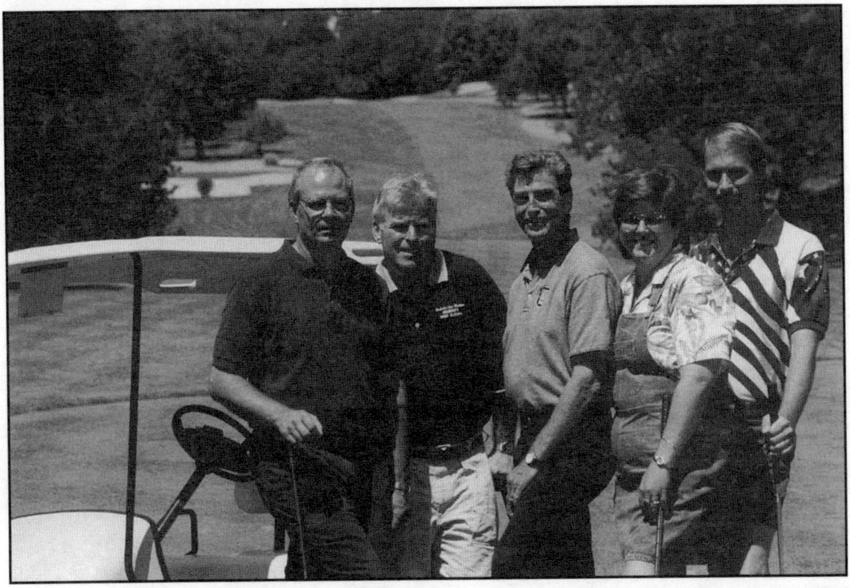

Promoting Organ and Tissue Donation

LifeCenter sponsored Champions for Life, a golf scramble, on September 24, 1999, at the Blue Ash Golf Course. The tournament raised more than $8,500. *Left to right:* David Lewis, LifeCenter's executive director; Dennis Janson, sports anchor at WCPO-TV in Cincinnati; Tom Starr, co-chairman; and Christine and Mike Frank, honorary co-chairpersons, whose two sons, James and Christopher, were killed in a traffic accident on I-275 in December 1998 and were organ and tissue donors.

Photograph © by Maslov Photography

This is a simple way to have a family discussion about organ and tissue donation. You and your family may be providing an opportunity for several other people you don't know to live or to improve the quality of their life. Saving a life is really very simple.

Donor cards and brochures are available at your local organ procurement organization. You may also indicate your intention to become an organ and tissue donor when you apply for or renew your driver's license.

Epilogue

At the University of Cincinnati Medical Center parking garage, there was an attendant who had a very unique perspective on life. It was refreshing and positive. Every time I'd see him I'd say, "Nice day today, isn't it?"

His reply: "Every day you're above ground is a good day." Too many people take life for granted and think that life owes them something. I take each day as it comes and live for the moment. I live every day as if it were my last. I enjoy life and I see the world with awe and amazement. Our time on this earth is short. When you get a second chance like I did, life is something to savor, as my wife, Debbie, likes to say.

I am thankful for each new day, every sunrise, and every sunset. I love my wife and the life we have made together. Debbie's love and faith is a constant inspiration. My mother, Adele, is probably the strongest and most faithful person I know. I don't tell her often enough how much I love her. I have a wonderful mother-in-law, Alma Pritchett. Debbie's grandmother, Christine Combs (Nan), died on February 2, 1999, at the age of 90.

Each morning and each evening I say a prayer for a 15-year-old young man I never knew and never met. His name was Brandon Burress. In death, he saved my life.

I say thank you to Dr. David Melvin, my cardiothoracic surgeon, and the entire transplant team; to Tom Tressler, former director of organ procurement at LifeCenter; and Tom Craycraft, former transplant coordinator and perfusionist, who helped recover my new heart. Both went out of their way to make me feel at ease when I started at LifeCenter. Tressler and I argued often about sports, mainly University of Cincinnati and Xavier basketball. He was in our wedding. He still is fun to be around, kind, generous and conscientious. He is now the regional director for the Make-a-Wish Foundation. That's a job where you can't have a bad day. I wish I saw him more often.

My job is great. I have many friends. I am happy. Life is good. High school students I lecture to on organ and tissue donation often ask me what my life expectancy is. I tell them I don't know. But even if I were to die tomorrow, I have had a wonderful life and a great second chance. As I write this, I am 45. The road of life for me has been rocky at times, but I'm still here. And that is what really matters.

If only one person who reads this book makes the decision to say "yes" to organ and tissue donation, then it has served its purpose, not only to inform but to offer someone else a second chance at life.

Index

Page numbers for illustrations are printed in *italics*.